WEIGHT LOSS

Culinary Solutions for Sustainable Weight Management

Aurora Dawn

CONTENTS

INTRODUCTION

Dear reader,

Welcome to "Weight Loss: Culinary Solutions for Sustainable Weight Management"! I am thrilled to have you join me on this journey towards healthier living through the transformative power of culinary solutions.

As we embark on this adventure together, I want you to know that you are not alone. Whether you're here seeking practical advice, culinary inspiration, or simply a supportive community to share your experiences with, you've come to the right place. Consider this book your virtual kitchen table—a place where you can gather with like-minded individuals who share your passion for delicious food and a desire to live a healthier, happier life.

Now, I'd like to invite you to take a moment to reflect on your own journey with weight management and cooking. What experiences have shaped your relationship with food? What aspirations do you have for your health and well-being? And most importantly, what do you hope to gain from reading this book?

Whether you're a seasoned chef or a kitchen novice, whether you've struggled with weight management for years or are just beginning your journey towards a healthier lifestyle, your voice and perspective are valued here. So, I encourage you to lean into the conversation, ask questions, share your insights, and connect with your fellow readers.

Together, let's explore the delicious possibilities that await us in the kitchen and discover the joy of nourishing our bodies and souls with every meal we create. Thank you for being a part of this community, and I look forward to sharing this journey with you.

Warmest regards,

Aurora Dawn

As I reflect on my own journey with weight management and my passion for cooking, one particular moment stands out vividly in my memory—a moment that profoundly shaped my perspective on food, health, and well-being.

Several years ago, I found myself standing in front of the mirror, feeling frustrated and defeated by the number staring back at me. Despite countless attempts to shed excess pounds through crash diets and intense exercise regimens, I seemed trapped in a cycle of temporary success followed by inevitable relapse.

It wasn't until I experienced a moment of clarity during a simple, yet profound, cooking session that everything changed. As I chopped fresh vegetables, stirred fragrant spices, and felt the warmth of the stove beneath my hands, I realized that my relationship with food was about so much more than just calories and portion sizes. It was about nourishment, creativity, and joy—a source of comfort and connection in a world often fraught with stress and uncertainty.

In that moment, I made a conscious decision to approach weight management from a new perspective—one grounded in the principles of balance, moderation, and mindfulness. Rather than viewing food as the enemy, I began to see it as a powerful ally in my quest for health and vitality.

This shift in mindset not only transformed the way I ate but also the way I lived. I started to prioritize fresh, whole ingredients over processed convenience foods, savoring each bite with gratitude and intention. I discovered the joy of experimenting with new flavors and cuisines, finding pleasure in the process of cooking and sharing meals with loved ones.

Through trial and error, perseverance, and a healthy dose of self-compassion, I gradually found my way to a healthier, happier version of myself. And along the way, I discovered a deep sense of fulfillment in helping others navigate their own journey towards better health and well-being through the transformative power of culinary solutions.

It is this journey—the highs and lows, the triumphs and challenges—that has fueled my passion for writing this book. I hope that by sharing my story, I can inspire and empower others to embrace a similar approach to weight management—one that celebrates the joy of cooking, the pleasures of the palate, and the profound connection between food and wellness.

So, as you embark on this journey with me, I invite you to open your heart and mind to the possibility of transformation. Together, let's explore the delicious possibilities that await us in the kitchen and discover the joy of nourishing our bodies and souls with every meal we create.

What sets *"Weight Loss: Culinary Solutions for Sustainable Weight Management"* apart from other books in the genre is its holistic approach to weight loss through culinary solutions. While many weight loss books focus solely on restrictive diets or intense exercise regimens, this book takes a different approach—one that celebrates the joy of cooking, the pleasures of the palate, and the transformative potential of culinary solutions.

One of the key distinguishing factors of this book is its innovative approach to recipes. Rather than offering a one-size-fits-all approach to weight loss, the recipes featured in this book are designed to be delicious, nutritious, and satisfying—making healthy eating a pleasure rather than a chore. From flavorful breakfasts to wholesome lunches, flavorful dinners, and guilt-free treats, each recipe is carefully crafted to support weight loss goals without sacrificing taste or enjoyment.

Additionally, this book goes beyond mere recipes to offer practical culinary strategies and techniques for reducing calorie intake, enhancing flavor, and fostering a deeper connection with food. Whether it's tips for ingredient substitutions, cooking methods, or meal planning, readers will find a wealth of actionable advice to help them achieve their weight loss goals in a sustainable and enjoyable way.

Furthermore, "Weight Loss: Culinary Solutions for Sustainable Management" distinguishes itself by its inclusion of expert insights and personal anecdotes. Drawing on the expertise of nutritionists, chefs, and wellness experts, as well as the author's own experiences and observations, this book offers a rich tapestry of wisdom and inspiration to guide readers on their weight loss journey. By combining evidence-based advice with real-life stories and practical tips, it provides a comprehensive roadmap for success that resonates with readers on a personal level.

In summary, what sets this book apart is its commitment to offering a holistic, sustainable approach to weight loss—one that celebrates the joy of cooking, nourishes the body and soul, and empowers readers to achieve lasting results. Whether you're a seasoned chef or a kitchen novice, whether you're embarking on your weight loss journey for the first time or seeking a fresh perspective on familiar territory, this book offers something truly unique and valuable.

By reading "Weight Loss: Culinary Solutions for Sustainable Management," you can expect to gain a wealth of valuable insights, practical tips, and inspiration to support you on your journey towards better health and well-being. Here's what you can look forward to:

Practical Tips and Advice: Discover a treasure trove of practical strategies and techniques for achieving sustainable weight loss through culinary solutions. From meal planning and portion control to ingredient substitutions and cooking methods, you'll learn how to make healthy eating a seamless and enjoyable part of your lifestyle.

Culinary Inspiration: Get ready to be inspired in the kitchen with a diverse array of delicious recipes that prove healthy eating can be both flavorful and satisfying. Whether you're craving a hearty breakfast, a nourishing lunch, a comforting dinner, or a guilt-free treat, you'll find plenty of culinary inspiration to tantalize your taste buds and keep you motivated on your weight loss journey.

Insights into the Science of Weight Loss: Gain a deeper understanding of the science behind weight loss, including the role of calories, metabolism, and nutrition. Learn how to harness the power of food to support your weight loss goals in a way that's backed by evidence and grounded in sound nutritional principles.

Sense of Empowerment and Motivation: Feel empowered to take control of your health and well-being as you explore the transformative potential of culinary solutions. Through expert advice, personal anecdotes, and real-life success stories, you'll be inspired to make positive changes in your life and embrace a healthier, happier lifestyle with confidence and enthusiasm.

Throughout the book, you'll find a comprehensive exploration of key themes and topics, including:

> ➤ The importance of building a strong foundation of healthy eating habits.

> ➤ Practical strategies for meal planning, preparation, and mindful eating.

> ➤ Delicious recipes for breakfasts, lunches, dinners, and snacks that support weight loss goals.

> ➤ Insights into the psychological and emotional aspects of eating behavior.

> ➤ Tips for overcoming challenges and staying motivated on your weight loss journey.

By providing a roadmap for success that's both practical and inspiring, "_Weight Loss: Culinary Solutions for Sustainable Weight Management_" offers readers a comprehensive guide to achieving their weight loss goals and embracing a healthier, happier lifestyle for the long term.

As you reach the end of this introduction, I want to leave you with a sense of excitement and empowerment as you embark on your journey towards better health and wellness. You've taken the first step by picking up this book, and now it's time to put what you've learned into action.

I encourage you to start by trying out one of the delicious recipes featured in the book. Whether it's a hearty breakfast to kickstart your day, a satisfying lunch to keep you fueled and focused, or a flavorful dinner to wind down after a long day, each recipe is designed to nourish your body and delight your taste buds.

Beyond the kitchen, I invite you to commit to making small, sustainable changes to your eating habits. Whether it's choosing whole, nutrient-rich foods over processed junk, practicing portion control, or simply being more mindful of what and how you eat, every step you take towards healthier eating brings you closer to your goals.

And finally, I encourage you to share your journey with others. Whether it's with friends, family, or fellow readers, sharing your experiences, challenges, and successes can be incredibly empowering and motivating. You never know who you might inspire along the way!

So, as you turn the page to start reading the first chapter, I invite you to keep an open mind and a curious spirit. And remember, you're not alone on this journey. Whether you're looking for additional resources, support, or just a friendly community to connect with, I'm here to help.

Thank you for joining me on this adventure towards better health and wellness. Here's to your success, your happiness, and your vibrant, nourished life ahead. Let's dive in together!

Warmest regards,

Aurora Dawn

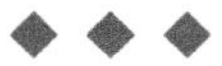

UNDERSTANDING WEIGHT LOSS

The Role Of Calories, Metabolism, And Nutrition

The science behind weight loss involves grasping the roles of calories, metabolism, and nutrition:

- ➢ Calories: Calories are units of energy derived from the food and beverages we consume. Weight loss fundamentally hinges on the concept of calorie balance – consuming fewer calories than the body expends. When the body experiences a calorie deficit, it turns to stored energy reserves (typically fat) for fuel, leading to weight loss over time. Conversely, a surplus of calories results in weight gain. Therefore, managing calorie intake is central to achieving and maintaining a healthy weight.

- ➢ Metabolism: Metabolism refers to the myriad chemical processes that occur within the body to sustain life. Basal metabolic rate (BMR) accounts for the majority of calories burned each day and is influenced by factors such as age, gender, body composition, and genetics. Physical activity and digestion also contribute to overall energy expenditure. While metabolism varies between individuals, it's important to note that certain factors, such as muscle mass and regular physical activity, can influence metabolic rate and contribute to weight management.

- ➢ Nutrition: Nutrition plays a pivotal role in weight loss, as the quality and composition of food directly impact overall health and metabolism. A balanced diet comprising adequate protein, healthy fats, complex carbohydrates, vitamins, and minerals is essential for supporting bodily functions and promoting satiety. By prioritizing nutrient-dense foods and mindful eating habits, individuals can optimize their nutrition intake and facilitate weight loss. Additionally, understanding portion sizes and practicing moderation can help maintain a healthy balance between calorie intake and expenditure.

In essence, weight loss is a multifaceted process that involves managing calorie intake, supporting metabolic function, and prioritizing nutrient-rich foods. By comprehending the science behind these key factors, individuals can make informed choices and adopt sustainable strategies to achieve their weight loss goals.

From my view when I started my weight loss journey, I knew I needed to understand the basics, and that meant wrapping my head around the concept of calories. Calories became my guiding star, the currency of my weight loss efforts.

I began to see calories not just as numbers on a label but as units of energy that fueled my body's every move. Every bite I took, every sip I drank, it all contributed to this energy balance equation. And if I wanted to see the numbers on the scale budge, I had to create a deficit – burning more calories than I consumed.

Tracking my calorie intake became a game-changer. It wasn't about deprivation or restriction but about making informed choices. I learned to swap out calorie-dense foods for more nutrient-rich options, finding satisfaction in nourishing my body while still staying within my calorie goals.

But it wasn't just about what I ate – it was also about how I moved. I discovered that every step I took, every workout I completed, was a chance to burn calories and tip the scales in my favor. Exercise became not just a means to an end but a way to celebrate what my body was capable of.

Of course, there were challenges along the way. There were days when I struggled to stay within my calorie limits, moments of frustration when the numbers on the scale didn't seem to budge. But through it all, I kept coming back to the simple truth: weight loss is a journey, and every calorie counts.

Now, as I continue on this path, I'm grateful for the lessons I've learned about calories and weight loss. They've become more than just numbers – they're a reminder of the power I have to shape my own health and well-being, one calorie at a time.

Weight loss boils down to a simple equation: consuming fewer calories than my body burns. It's like managing a budget – if I spend more money than I earn, I end up in debt. Similarly, if I eat more calories than my body needs, those excess calories get stored as fat, leading to weight gain.

Understanding this concept was a game-changer for me. It meant I didn't have to follow complicated diets or cut out entire food groups. Instead, I could focus on making small, sustainable changes to my eating habits and lifestyle.

Tracking my calorie intake was key. It gave me a clear picture of how much I was eating and where I could make adjustments. I started paying more attention to portion sizes, choosing nutrient-dense foods, and cutting back on empty calories like sugary snacks and sodas.

But it wasn't just about cutting calories – it was also about burning more through exercise and physical activity. I found activities I enjoyed, whether it was going for a run, taking a dance class, or simply going for a walk in the park. Not only did it help me burn calories, but it also boosted my mood and energy levels.

There were challenges along the way. There were days when I slipped up or felt frustrated with my progress. But I reminded myself that every little bit counts – every healthy meal, every workout, every step taken towards my goals.

Now, as I continue on my journey, I know that achieving a calorie deficit is the foundation of my success. It's not about perfection or deprivation but about finding a balance that works for me – one that allows me to enjoy life while still making progress towards my weight loss goals.

From my own experience, understanding the role of metabolism in weight management has been crucial on my journey to a healthier lifestyle.

Metabolism isn't just some mysterious force – it's the engine that powers everything our bodies do, from breathing to digesting food to exercising. And when it comes to weight management, metabolism plays a key role in determining how efficiently we burn calories and how quickly we lose or gain weight.

For me, learning about metabolism was like unlocking the secret to why some people seem to be able to eat whatever they want without gaining weight, while others struggle to lose even a few pounds. I realized that factors like age, gender, genetics, and muscle mass all play a role in determining our metabolic rate.

But here's the thing – while we can't change our genetics, we can definitely influence our metabolism through lifestyle choices. I discovered that regular exercise, especially strength training, can help boost metabolism by building lean muscle mass. And by eating a balanced diet with plenty of protein, healthy fats, and complex carbohydrates, I could keep my metabolism firing on all cylinders.

Of course, there are no quick fixes when it comes to metabolism. Crash diets and extreme exercise regimens might give you temporary results, but they can also slow down your metabolism and make it even harder to lose weight in the long run. That's why I've learned to focus on sustainable habits that support a healthy metabolism, like getting enough sleep, managing stress, and staying hydrated.

In the end, understanding the role of metabolism in weight management has been empowering for me. It's helped me see that I have more control over my body than I ever thought possible, and that by making smart choices and listening to my body, I can achieve my weight loss goals while still feeling strong, healthy, and energized.

Myth: Crash diets are effective for long-term weight loss.

Crash diets often promise quick results, but the reality is far from sustainable. While they may lead to rapid weight loss initially, crash diets are typically unsustainable and can have detrimental effects on overall health. Here's a breakdown of why:

> Nutrient Deficiencies: Crash diets often severely restrict food intake, which can lead to nutrient deficiencies. Essential vitamins, minerals, and other nutrients are necessary for maintaining optimal health and supporting bodily functions. By depriving the body of essential nutrients, crash diets can increase the risk of nutritional deficiencies and related

health problems.

➤ Muscle Loss: Rapid weight loss from crash diets often comes from water weight and muscle mass, rather than fat loss. Muscle loss is particularly problematic because muscle tissue is metabolically active and helps to support a healthy metabolism. Losing muscle mass can lead to a slower metabolism and difficulty maintaining weight loss in the long term.

➤ Metabolic Slowdown: Crash diets can also lead to a slowdown in metabolism, making it harder to lose weight and easier to regain lost weight once the diet is over. The body may adapt to the reduced calorie intake by conserving energy and burning fewer calories, making weight loss more challenging.

In contrast, long-term success in weight management requires a balanced, sustainable approach to eating. This involves consuming a variety of nutrient-rich foods in appropriate portions, staying physically active, and adopting healthy lifestyle habits.

Myth: Carbohydrates are the enemy and should be avoided for weight loss.

Carbohydrates are a vital source of energy and essential nutrients that play a crucial role in a balanced diet. While it's true that refined carbohydrates should be limited due to their lower nutrient content and potential negative impact on blood sugar levels, it's essential to recognize the importance of incorporating whole grains, fruits, and vegetables into a healthy eating plan.

Here's why carbohydrates, particularly from whole food sources, are beneficial for health:

➤ Energy Source: Carbohydrates are the body's primary source of energy, providing fuel for physical activity, brain function, and everyday tasks. Whole grains, fruits, and vegetables supply complex carbohydrates, which are broken down more slowly in the body, providing sustained energy throughout the day.

➤ Nutrient Density: Whole grains, fruits, and vegetables are rich in essential nutrients such as vitamins, minerals, fiber, and antioxidants. These nutrients play critical roles in supporting overall health, including immune function, digestion, and heart health.

➤ Fiber Content: Whole grains, fruits, and vegetables are excellent sources of dietary fiber, which is essential for digestive health, promoting satiety, and regulating blood sugar levels. High-fiber foods can help prevent constipation, control hunger, and support weight management.

➤ Disease Prevention: Consuming a diet rich in whole grains, fruits, and vegetables has been linked to a reduced risk of chronic diseases such as heart disease, diabetes, and certain cancers. The nutrients and phytochemicals found in these foods have protective effects on overall health and well-being.

Overall, while it's important to be mindful of the types and amounts of carbohydrates consumed, whole grains, fruits, and vegetables are nutritious staples that should be included as part of a healthy diet. By focusing on nutrient-dense, whole food sources of carbohydrates, individuals can support their overall health and well-being while enjoying a variety of delicious and satisfying meals.

There are quite a few misconceptions and myths about metabolism that I've encountered on my weight loss journey. One of the biggest ones is the idea that certain foods or supplements have the magical power to dramatically boost metabolism.

I used to believe that if I just ate enough spicy foods or drank enough green tea, I could rev up my metabolism and melt away the pounds. But the truth is, while some foods and drinks may have a minor impact on metabolism, there's no magic bullet when it comes to speeding it up.

Sure, spicy foods like chili peppers contain compounds like capsaicin that can temporarily increase metabolism, but the effect is pretty small and short-lived. And while caffeine found in green tea and coffee can slightly boost metabolism, relying on it as a weight loss solution isn't sustainable or healthy in the long run.

Another common misconception is that certain supplements or pills can supercharge metabolism and lead to rapid weight loss. I used to see ads for "metabolism-boosting" supplements everywhere, promising to help me shed pounds effortlessly. But the reality is that most of these supplements are unregulated and often ineffective – and some can even be dangerous.

Instead of falling for these myths, I've learned to focus on more practical strategies for supporting a healthy metabolism. Eating a balanced diet with plenty of protein, healthy fats, and complex carbohydrates helps keep my metabolism running smoothly. And regular exercise, especially strength training, helps build lean muscle mass, which can boost metabolism over time.

Overall, I've come to realize that while metabolism is important for weight management, it's not something that can be dramatically altered with a special food or supplement. Instead, it's about making smart, sustainable lifestyle choices that support overall health and well-being.

I've come to understand just how much factors like age, gender, body composition, and physical activity level can influence our metabolic rate – and ultimately, our ability to manage our weight.

Age is something we all experience, and with it comes changes in our metabolism. As we get older, our metabolism tends to slow down. It's like our body's engine isn't running as fast as it used to. This can be frustrating, but it's a natural part of aging, and something we can work with by making adjustments to our lifestyle and diet.

Gender also plays a role in metabolism. Men and women have different hormonal profiles and body compositions, which can affect how many calories we burn at rest. Men tend to have more muscle mass, which means they typically have a higher metabolic rate compared to women. Understanding these differences has helped me tailor my approach to weight management to better suit my own body.

Speaking of body composition, it's another key factor in metabolism. Muscle tissue burns more calories than fat tissue, even when we're at rest. So, the more muscle you have, the higher your metabolic rate is likely to be. This is why strength training and building muscle through exercise are so important for maintaining a healthy metabolism.

And then there's physical activity level. How active we are throughout the day – whether it's going for a run, walking the dog, or just moving around the house – can have a big impact on our metabolic rate. Regular exercise not only burns calories during workouts but can also boost our metabolism for hours afterward.

Understanding how these factors influence metabolism has been incredibly empowering for me. It's helped me take a more personalized approach to weight management, focusing on strategies that work best for my own body and lifestyle. By paying attention to age, gender, body composition, and physical activity level, I've been able to support my metabolism and achieve my health and fitness goals more effectively.

To realize just how critical nutrition is when it comes to achieving sustainable weight loss. It's not just about cutting calories or following the latest fad diet – it's about nourishing your body with the right foods to support your health and well-being.

For me, sustainable weight loss isn't about deprivation or going on extreme diets. It's about making smart, informed choices about what I eat and finding a balance that works for me. That means focusing on nutrient-dense foods that provide essential vitamins, minerals, and other nutrients my body needs to thrive.

I've learned to prioritize whole, unprocessed foods like fruits, vegetables, lean proteins, and whole grains. These foods not only help me feel satisfied and energized, but they also support my weight loss goals by providing the nutrients my body needs to function optimally.

At the same time, I've become more mindful of my portion sizes and eating habits. I've learned to listen to my body's hunger and fullness cues and to eat mindfully, savoring each bite and enjoying the experience of eating.

But it's not just about what I eat – it's also about how I eat. I've learned to be more mindful of my eating habits, paying attention to when and why I eat and making conscious choices about my food intake.

And perhaps most importantly, I've come to realize that sustainable weight loss is about more than just the number on the scale. It's about feeling good in my body, having energy to do the things I love, and nourishing myself from the inside out.

To appreciate the immense importance of balanced nutrition in supporting overall health and well-being. It's not just about counting calories or focusing on specific food groups – it's about nourishing your body with a variety of nutrients that it needs to thrive.

One of the key components of balanced nutrition is adequate protein. Protein is essential for building and repairing tissues, supporting muscle growth, and regulating hormones. Including sources of lean protein like chicken, fish, tofu, beans, and lentils in my diet has helped me feel more satisfied and energized throughout the day.

Healthy fats are another crucial part of balanced nutrition. Contrary to popular belief, fats are not the enemy – in fact, they play a vital role in brain health, hormone production, and absorption of fat-soluble vitamins. Incorporating sources of healthy fats like avocados, nuts, seeds, and olive oil into my meals has not only improved my overall health but also helped me feel more satisfied and satisfied.

Complex carbohydrates are essential for providing the body with long-lasting energy and supporting optimal brain function. Unlike simple carbohydrates, which can cause blood sugar spikes and crashes, complex carbohydrates like whole grains, fruits, and vegetables provide a steady source of fuel that keeps me feeling energized and focused throughout the day.

Of course, balanced nutrition isn't just about macronutrients – it's also about ensuring an adequate intake of vitamins and minerals. These micronutrients play critical roles in immune function, bone health, and countless other physiological processes. Eating a diverse array of fruits, vegetables, whole grains, and lean proteins ensures that I get the vitamins and minerals my body needs to function at its best.

Overall, balanced nutrition is the cornerstone of a healthy lifestyle. By prioritizing adequate protein, healthy fats, complex carbohydrates, vitamins, and minerals in my diet, I've been able to support my overall health and well-being, feel more energized and focused, and achieve my weight loss goals in a sustainable way.

It's become clear that there's no shortage of dietary trends and fads out there promising quick fixes and miraculous results. But as enticing as these trends may seem, I've learned to approach them with a healthy dose of skepticism and a focus on what truly matters: a varied and nutrient-dense diet.

One of the most pervasive myths surrounding dietary trends is the idea that cutting out entire food groups is necessary for success. Whether it's eliminating carbs, fats, or even entire food categories like gluten or dairy, these restrictive approaches can be both unnecessary and potentially harmful. Our bodies need a wide variety of nutrients to function optimally, and cutting out entire food groups can lead to nutrient deficiencies and imbalances.

Another common myth is the belief that certain foods or ingredients are inherently "good" or "bad" for you. Whether it's demonizing carbs, vilifying fats, or glorifying superfoods, these black-and-white approaches oversimplify the complex relationship between food and health. In reality, it's the overall pattern of eating that matters most – focusing on a diverse array of nutrient-rich foods rather than fixating on individual ingredients.

Then there's the misconception that dietary supplements or quick-fix solutions can make up for poor eating habits. Whether it's detox teas, fat-burning pills, or meal replacement shakes, these products often promise dramatic results with little effort. But the truth is, there's no substitute for a balanced diet rich in whole, unprocessed foods. Supplements can be helpful in certain situations, but they should never be relied upon as a substitute for a healthy diet.

I've learned that many popular diets and trends promise quick fixes, but they often overlook the importance of a balanced and nutritious diet.

Myth 1: Cutting out entire food groups is necessary for success.

Reality: Our bodies need a variety of nutrients, so cutting out entire food groups can lead to deficiencies.

Myth 2: Some foods are inherently "good" or "bad."

Reality: It's the overall pattern of eating that matters most, so focus on a diverse array of nutrient-rich foods.

Myth 3: Dietary supplements can make up for poor eating habits.

Reality: While supplements can be helpful, they're not a substitute for a healthy diet rich in whole foods.

By understanding these myths and prioritizing a balanced diet full of fruits, vegetables, lean proteins, whole grains, and healthy fats, I've been able to adopt a sustainable approach to eating that supports my long-term health and well-being.

◆ ◆ ◆

COMMON MISCONCEPTIONS AND MYTHS:

Navigating the myriad of misconceptions and myths surrounding weight loss has been a journey in itself. Here are some of the most pervasive ones I've encountered:

Myth 1: Crash diets are the quickest way to lose weight.

Reality: Crash diets, characterized by severe calorie restriction or extreme dietary limitations, may yield rapid weight loss initially. However, this weight loss is often unsustainable and can lead to a host of negative health consequences. These diets typically fail to address long-term lifestyle changes and may result in nutrient deficiencies, muscle loss, and metabolic slowdown. In the end, sustainable weight loss requires a balanced approach that focuses on gradual, healthy changes to eating habits and lifestyle.

Myth 2: Certain foods or supplements can magically melt away fat.

Reality: The weight loss industry is rife with claims of "miracle" foods, supplements, or ingredients purported to accelerate fat loss without the need for diet or exercise. However, these claims are often unsupported by scientific evidence. While some foods or supplements may have modest effects on metabolism or appetite regulation, there is no single food or supplement that can replace the fundamental principles of calorie balance and healthy eating. Sustainable weight loss requires a comprehensive approach that includes balanced nutrition, regular physical activity, and behavior modification.

Myth 3: You have to starve yourself to lose weight.

Reality: The idea that severe calorie restriction is necessary for weight loss is a common misconception. In reality, overly restrictive diets are not only unsustainable but also counterproductive. Severely restricting calories can slow down metabolism, increase the risk of nutrient deficiencies, and lead to loss of muscle mass. Moreover, extreme hunger and deprivation are often followed by periods of overeating or bingeing, sabotaging weight loss efforts in the long run. Instead, sustainable weight loss involves creating a moderate calorie deficit through a balanced diet that includes a variety of nutrient-dense foods and regular physical activity.

Let's address these myths with evidence-based insights:

Myth: Cutting out entire food groups is necessary for success.

Reality: In my experience, I've learned that cutting out entire food groups is not only unnecessary but can also be detrimental to overall health. Each food group offers unique nutrients that are essential for our bodies to function optimally. For example, carbohydrates provide energy, protein supports muscle repair and growth, and fats are crucial for hormone regulation and nutrient absorption. By including a variety of foods from all food groups in my diet, I ensure that I'm getting a wide range of nutrients necessary for good health.

Myth: Certain foods can magically melt away fat.

Reality: While it's tempting to believe in the power of "fat-burning" foods or ingredients, the truth is that weight loss is a complex process that requires more than just eating specific foods. No single food has the ability to target fat loss in specific areas of the body. Sustainable weight loss is achieved through a combination of factors, including creating a calorie deficit, regular exercise, and adopting healthy eating habits. Instead of focusing on specific "fat-burning" foods, I prioritize a balanced diet rich in whole, unprocessed foods that nourish my body and support overall health.

Understanding the role of genetics, hormones, and other factors in weight loss has been enlightening and has helped me approach weight management with a more holistic mindset.

Firstly, "genetics" play a significant role in determining our body weight and how we respond to different diets and exercises. I've come to realize that our genetic makeup can influence our metabolism, fat distribution, and even our hunger and satiety signals. This means that while some people may lose weight easily with certain diets or exercise routines, others may struggle despite their best efforts. Recognizing the genetic component has helped me be more patient and compassionate with myself, understanding that weight management is not a one-size-fits-all process.

"Hormones" are another crucial factor. Hormones like insulin, cortisol, leptin, and ghrelin have a profound impact on our appetite, metabolism, and fat storage. For instance, I've learned that high stress levels can increase cortisol, which may lead to weight gain, especially around the abdomen. Similarly, imbalances in insulin can affect how our body stores fat and uses glucose for energy. Understanding the role of hormones has led me to focus not just on diet and exercise, but also on managing stress, getting adequate sleep, and maintaining a balanced lifestyle to support hormonal health.

There are also other factors like "sleep, stress, and mental health" that significantly influence weight management. For example, poor sleep can disrupt hormones like leptin and ghrelin, which regulate hunger and fullness, leading to increased appetite and potential weight gain. Stress, on the other hand, can trigger emotional eating or cravings for high-calorie, sugary foods. By addressing these aspects of my life, I've found that I'm better able to manage my weight.

Additionally, "environmental factors" such as access to healthy foods, socioeconomic status, and even the people we surround ourselves with can influence our weight. Living in an environment where healthy food options are scarce or where there's a lack of support for healthy living can make weight management more challenging.

Recognizing that successful weight management is a complex interplay of these various factors has been incredibly empowering. It has taught me that while diet and exercise are important, they are just pieces of a larger puzzle. By considering genetics, hormones, sleep, stress, and environment, I can create a more comprehensive and realistic approach to achieving and maintaining a healthy weight. This holistic understanding has allowed me to set more achievable goals, be kinder to myself, and find strategies that work specifically for my body and lifestyle.

From my own journey, I've found that empowering myself with knowledge and developing a realistic, sustainable approach to weight loss has been transformative. Here's how I approached it, and how you can too:

1. Educate Yourself:

Understanding the basics of nutrition, metabolism, and the factors influencing weight loss is crucial. For me, learning about how my body works helped demystify the process and debunk many myths. I realized that weight loss isn't just about calories in versus calories out; it's about nourishing my body with the right nutrients, understanding my metabolic rate, and considering factors like genetics and hormones.

2. Set Realistic Goals:

One of the biggest lessons I learned was to set achievable, realistic goals. Instead of aiming for rapid weight loss, I focused on gradual changes that I could maintain over the long term. This approach helped me avoid the frustration and disappointment that often come with unrealistic expectations.

3. Focus on Balanced Nutrition:

I started prioritizing a balanced diet rich in whole foods. Instead of cutting out entire food groups, I embraced a variety of nutrients: adequate protein for muscle maintenance, healthy fats for hormone balance, complex carbohydrates for energy, and plenty of vitamins and minerals from fruits and vegetables. This not only supported my weight loss but also improved my overall health and well-being.

4. Incorporate Regular Physical Activity:

Exercise became an integral part of my routine, not just for burning calories but for building strength, improving mood, and boosting metabolism. Finding activities I enjoy, like hiking and swimming, made it easier to stay consistent and motivated.

5. Understand and Manage Hormones and Stress:

Recognizing the impact of hormones and stress on weight was a game-changer. I began to focus on stress management techniques like yoga, meditation, and ensuring adequate sleep. This holistic approach helped balance my hormones, reduce emotional eating, and improve my overall quality of life.

6. Be Kind to Yourself:

Self-compassion and patience are essential. I learned to celebrate small victories and not to be too hard on myself during setbacks. Weight loss is a journey with ups and downs, and it's important to stay positive and persistent.

7. Seek Support and Community:

Surrounding myself with supportive friends, family, and communities helped me stay motivated and accountable. Sharing experiences, challenges, and successes with others who are on similar journeys can be incredibly empowering.

By making informed choices and focusing on a balanced, realistic approach, I found a path to sustainable weight loss that fits my lifestyle. It's not about perfection but about progress and maintaining a healthy relationship with food and my body.

THE FOUNDATION OF HEALTHY EATING

Building a strong foundation of healthy eating habits has been the cornerstone of my weight loss journey. This foundation isn't about strict diets or temporary changes, but about creating lasting habits that support long-term health and well-being. Here's how I've focused on establishing this strong foundation:

1. Prioritize Whole Foods:

I made a conscious effort to incorporate more whole, unprocessed foods into my diet. These foods, such as fruits, vegetables, lean proteins, whole grains, and healthy fats, are packed with essential nutrients and are far more satisfying than processed options. By filling my plate with these nutrient-dense foods, I provide my body with the fuel it needs to function optimally.

2. Practice Mindful Eating:

Learning to eat mindfully has been a game-changer. I started paying attention to my hunger and fullness cues, savoring each bite, and avoiding distractions while eating. This practice has helped me enjoy my meals more and prevent overeating, making it easier to maintain a healthy weight.

3. Plan and Prepare Meals:

Planning and preparing meals in advance has helped me stay on track with my healthy eating goals. By cooking at home and preparing my meals ahead of time, I have better control over the ingredients and portion sizes. This also helps me avoid the temptation of unhealthy convenience foods when I'm busy or tired.

4. Balance Macronutrients:

Ensuring that my meals are balanced with adequate protein, healthy fats, and complex carbohydrates has been crucial. Protein keeps me full and supports muscle maintenance, healthy fats are essential for hormone production and nutrient absorption, and complex carbs provide sustained energy. This balance helps me feel satisfied and energized throughout the day.

5. Stay Hydrated:

Drinking plenty of water is a simple yet effective habit that supports overall health and aids in weight management. Staying hydrated helps regulate appetite, supports metabolism, and keeps my body functioning properly. I've made it a habit to carry a water bottle with me and sip water throughout the day.

6. Limit Added Sugars and Processed Foods:

Reducing my intake of added sugars and processed foods has made a significant difference in my health. These foods are often high in empty calories and low in nutrients, leading to energy crashes and increased cravings. By focusing on whole foods and minimizing sugary snacks and beverages, I've been able to maintain more stable energy levels and better control my appetite.

7. Be Consistent, Not Perfect:

Embracing consistency over perfection has been key. There will always be occasional indulgences and setbacks, but what matters most is maintaining healthy habits most of the time. Allowing myself flexibility and enjoying treats in moderation has made it easier to stick to my healthy eating habits long-term.

Building a strong foundation of healthy eating habits has empowered me to take control of my health and achieve sustainable weight loss. These habits are not about restriction but about nourishing my body, enjoying my food, and creating a balanced lifestyle that I can maintain for the long haul.

Understanding and applying the principles of balanced nutrition, portion control, and mindful eating has been essential for achieving and maintaining a healthy weight. Here's how I've incorporated these principles into my daily life:

Balanced Nutrition

Balanced nutrition is the foundation of a healthy diet. It involves consuming a variety of foods that provide all the essential nutrients your body needs to function optimally.

- ➢ Macronutrients: I focus on including the right proportions of macronutrients in my meals: proteins, fats, and carbohydrates. Proteins are vital for muscle repair and growth, healthy fats are essential for hormone production and nutrient absorption, and carbohydrates provide the energy needed for daily activities. For example, a typical meal might include grilled chicken (protein), avocado (healthy fat), and quinoa (complex carbohydrate).

- ➢ Micronutrients: Vitamins and minerals are equally important. By eating a wide range of fruits and vegetables, I ensure I get the necessary vitamins and minerals that support various bodily functions and prevent deficiencies.

- ➢ Variety and Color: Including a variety of colorful foods not only makes meals more appealing but also ensures a broader intake of nutrients. Each color in fruits and vegetables often represents different phytonutrients and antioxidants, which are beneficial for health.

Portion Control

Portion control is crucial for maintaining a healthy weight. It helps prevent overeating and ensures that you consume the right amount of calories to meet your energy needs without excess.

- ➤ Understanding Serving Sizes: I educated myself on what constitutes a proper serving size for different food groups. This helped me avoid unintentional overeating, especially with calorie-dense foods like nuts and cheese.

- ➤ Using Smaller Plates: A simple trick that has worked for me is using smaller plates and bowls. This creates the illusion of a fuller plate with smaller portions, which can help reduce overall calorie intake.

- ➤ Listening to Hunger Cues: Instead of eating until I'm overly full, I learned to recognize my body's hunger and fullness signals. Eating slowly and paying attention to how I feel during meals has helped me stop eating when I'm satisfied, not stuffed.

Mindful Eating

Mindful eating is about being present and fully engaged with the eating experience. This practice has transformed my relationship with food and helped me make more conscious choices.

- ➤ Eliminating Distractions: I try to eat without distractions like TV or smartphones. This allows me to focus on the flavors, textures, and enjoyment of my food, making me more aware of what and how much I'm eating.

- ➤ Savoring Each Bite: By taking the time to savor each bite, I've found that I enjoy my meals more and feel satisfied with less food. This also helps in slowing down the eating process, which is beneficial for digestion and recognizing fullness signals.

- ➤ Reflecting on Food Choices: Mindful eating encourages me to think about why I'm eating. Am I truly hungry, or am I eating out of boredom, stress, or habit? This self-awareness helps me make healthier choices and avoid emotional eating.

Incorporating the principles of balanced nutrition, portion control, and mindful eating into my lifestyle has been a game-changer. It has not only helped me manage my weight more effectively but also improved my overall relationship with food.

◆ ◆ ◆

CULINARY STRATEGIES
FOR WEIGHT LOSS

Reducing calorie intake without sacrificing flavor is entirely achievable with a few practical culinary strategies and techniques. Here are some approaches that have worked well for me:

Culinary Strategies and Techniques

1. Use Herbs and Spices:

One of the best ways to enhance the flavor of your dishes without adding extra calories is by using herbs and spices. Fresh herbs like basil, cilantro, and parsley, as well as spices like cumin, paprika, and turmeric, can add depth and complexity to your meals. For instance, I love adding a sprinkle of smoked paprika to roasted vegetables or fresh cilantro to salads and soups.

2. Incorporate Low-Calorie Flavor Boosters:

Ingredients like garlic, ginger, lemon zest, and lime juice can significantly enhance the taste of your food without adding many calories. I often use lemon zest and juice to brighten up a salad or grilled chicken. A splash of vinegar or a dash of hot sauce can also add a flavorful punch to dishes.

3. Opt for Cooking Methods that Require Less Fat:

Cooking methods like grilling, baking, steaming, and poaching can help reduce the amount of added fats needed for cooking. For example, I often grill my vegetables and proteins instead of frying them. This method not only reduces calories but also adds a delicious smoky flavor.

4.Use Healthy Substitutes:

Substituting high-calorie ingredients with healthier, lower-calorie alternatives can make a big difference. For instance, I use Greek yogurt instead of sour cream or mayonnaise in dressings and dips. Instead of heavy cream, I use pureed cauliflower or cashews to add creaminess to soups and sauces.

5. Increase Vegetable Content:

Vegetables are low in calories and high in nutrients and fiber, making them an excellent way to bulk up your meals. I often add extra vegetables to my pasta dishes, casseroles, and stir-fries. Spiralized zucchini or carrots can be a great substitute for pasta, reducing calorie intake while increasing vegetable consumption.

6. Control Portions with Smart Serving Techniques:

Using smaller plates and bowls can help control portion sizes and reduce calorie intake. Additionally, I measure out serving sizes instead of eating directly from the package, which helps prevent overeating. For example, I portion out snacks like nuts or chips into small bowls instead of eating from the bag.

7. Be Mindful of Sauces and Dressings:

Many sauces and dressings are high in calories, so I've learned to be mindful of how much I use. I make my own vinaigrettes using a small amount of olive oil mixed with vinegar or lemon juice, mustard, and herbs. When using store-bought dressings, I choose lighter options and use them sparingly.

8. Choose Lean Proteins:

Opting for lean proteins such as chicken breast, turkey, fish, and plant-based proteins like beans and legumes can help reduce calorie intake. I also trim visible fat from meats and remove the skin from poultry before cooking.

9. Incorporate Whole Grains:

Whole grains like quinoa, brown rice, and oats are more filling and nutritious than refined grains. They also have a lower glycemic index, which can help control appetite and reduce calorie intake. I've found that incorporating these grains into my meals keeps me satisfied for longer.

10. Hydrate with Water-Rich Foods:

Including water-rich foods like cucumbers, tomatoes, watermelon, and leafy greens in meals can help increase fullness and reduce overall calorie intake. These foods are refreshing, hydrating, and low in calories, making them perfect for snacks and meal additions.

11. Batch Cook and Meal Prep:

Planning and preparing meals in advance can help control portions and reduce the temptation to eat high-calorie convenience foods. I often spend a few hours on the weekend batch cooking and portioning out meals for the week. This way, I have healthy, ready-to-eat options that help me stay on track.

12. Experiment with Low-Calorie Ingredients:

Ingredients like zucchini noodles (zoodles), cauliflower rice, and spaghetti squash can replace higher-calorie counterparts like pasta and rice. I frequently use cauliflower rice in stir-fries or as a base for grain bowls, which significantly cuts down on calories while still providing a satisfying meal.

13. Use Cooking Sprays Instead of Oil:

While cooking sprays may not entirely replace the flavor and richness of oil, they can significantly reduce the amount of fat and calories in a dish. I use a light spray to coat pans before sautéing vegetables or proteins, ensuring they don't stick without adding excess calories.

14. Increase Fiber Intake:

Foods high in fiber, such as beans, lentils, whole grains, fruits, and vegetables, can help you feel fuller for longer. I incorporate fiber-rich foods into my meals by adding beans to salads, soups, and stews, and choosing whole fruits over fruit juices.

15. Make Healthy Swaps for High-Calorie Ingredients:

Simple swaps can make a big difference in reducing calorie intake. For example, I use mashed avocado in place of butter on toast, swap out sour cream for Greek yogurt in recipes, and use unsweetened applesauce as a substitute for oil or butter in baking.

16. Watch Your Beverages:

Calories from beverages can add up quickly. I've made a habit of drinking water, herbal teas, and black coffee instead of sugary drinks and sodas. If I want something more flavorful, I infuse my water with slices of lemon, cucumber, or berries.

17. Practice Mindful Portion Control for Snacks:

Instead of eating directly from a large bag or box, I portion out snacks into small containers. This helps me enjoy my favorite treats without overeating. For example, I measure a serving of nuts or popcorn and put it in a small bowl, which makes it easier to stick to a reasonable portion size.

18. Utilize Healthy Cooking Methods:

Methods like steaming, grilling, roasting, and baking can reduce the need for added fats compared to frying. I often steam vegetables to retain their nutrients, grill lean meats for a smoky flavor without added fat, and roast vegetables with just a touch of olive oil for a delicious caramelized taste.

19. Incorporate More Plant-Based Meals:

Plant-based meals tend to be lower in calories and high in nutrients. I've found that incorporating more vegetarian and vegan meals into my diet helps reduce calorie intake while providing a variety of vitamins, minerals, and antioxidants. For instance, a hearty lentil soup or a chickpea salad can be both satisfying and nutritious.

20. Limit High-Calorie Condiments:

Many condiments are high in sugar, fat, and calories. I choose healthier alternatives like mustard, salsa, or homemade dressings made with yogurt or vinegar. When I do use higher-calorie condiments like mayonnaise or ketchup, I use them sparingly.

21. Choose Satiating Foods:

Foods with a high satiety index, such as eggs, oats, potatoes, and lean meats, help keep me full longer. Including these foods in my meals helps me stay satisfied and reduces the likelihood of overeating. For example, starting my day with a bowl of oatmeal topped with berries and a boiled egg keeps me full until lunchtime.

22. Emphasize Protein-Rich Snacks:

Snacking on protein-rich foods like Greek yogurt, cottage cheese, nuts, or hummus with vegetables can help curb hunger between meals. I've found that these snacks provide lasting energy and keep my appetite in check.

◆ ◆ ◆

TIPS FOR INGREDIENT SUBSTITUTIONS, COOKING METHODS, AND FLAVOR ENHANCEMENT

Ingredient Substitutions

1. Greek Yogurt for Sour Cream or Mayonnaise:

Greek yogurt is a great substitute for sour cream or mayonnaise in dips, dressings, and sandwiches. It's lower in calories and fat, but still creamy and tangy.

2. Cauliflower for Rice or Potatoes:

Cauliflower can be used as a low-calorie alternative to rice or mashed potatoes. Simply pulse cauliflower in a food processor to create "rice" or steam and mash it for a creamy potato substitute.

3. Zucchini Noodles (Zoodles) for Pasta:

Using a spiralizer, you can create noodles from zucchini. Zoodles are a low-carb and low-calorie substitute for traditional pasta, perfect for dishes like spaghetti or stir-fries.

4. Avocado for Butter:

Avocado can replace butter in baked goods and spreads. It provides healthy fats and a creamy texture, reducing saturated fat intake.

5. Mashed Banana or Applesauce for Sugar:

Mashed banana or unsweetened applesauce can be used to sweeten baked goods naturally, cutting down on added sugars while adding moisture.

6. Nut Butters for Butter or Oil in Baking:

Replacing butter or oil with nut butters like almond or peanut butter adds protein and healthy fats to baked goods, making them more nutritious.

7. Whole Wheat Flour for White Flour:

Whole wheat flour has more fiber and nutrients than white flour. It can be used in equal parts or mixed with white flour to add a nutritional boost to baked goods.

Cooking Methods

1. Grilling:

Grilling adds a smoky flavor to meats, vegetables, and fruits without needing much added fat. It's a healthy alternative to frying and enhances the natural flavors of foods.

2. Steaming:

Steaming preserves the nutrients in vegetables and seafood while maintaining their natural flavors. It's a low-fat cooking method that keeps foods light and healthy.

3. Baking:

Baking is a versatile method that can be used for meats, vegetables, and baked goods. Using parchment paper or a silicone mat reduces the need for added fats.

4. Roasting:

Roasting caramelizes the natural sugars in vegetables and meats, enhancing their flavors. Using a small amount of olive oil can create a delicious, crispy texture without excess calories.

5. Poaching:

Poaching involves gently cooking food in simmering liquid. It's perfect for delicate items like fish or eggs and doesn't require added fats.

6. Sautéing with Broth:

Instead of using oil or butter, I often sauté vegetables in low-sodium broth. This method adds flavor without the extra calories from fats.

Flavor Enhancement

1. Herbs and Spices:

Fresh and dried herbs and spices can add depth and complexity to dishes without extra calories. Experiment with basil, cilantro, rosemary, thyme, cumin, paprika, and turmeric.

2. Citrus Zest and Juice:

Lemon, lime, and orange zest add a bright, fresh flavor to dishes. Citrus juice can be used to marinate meats, enhance dressings, or finish cooked vegetables.

3. Vinegars:

Vinegars such as balsamic, apple cider, and red wine vinegar add tanginess and depth to salads, marinades, and cooked dishes.

4. Garlic and Onions:

These aromatic vegetables add a robust flavor base to many dishes. Roasting or caramelizing them can enhance their sweetness and add richness to meals.

5. Low-Sodium Soy Sauce or Tamari:

These add a savory umami flavor to stir-fries, marinades, and sauces. Opting for low-sodium versions helps control salt intake.

6. Nutritional Yeast:

This can add a cheesy, nutty flavor to dishes. It's great for sprinkling on popcorn, adding to sauces, or mixing into pasta dishes for a boost of flavor and nutrients.

7. Infused Oils:

Using small amounts of infused oils like garlic or chili oil can add a burst of flavor to dishes. A little goes a long way, so you can keep calorie intake low.

8. Homemade Broths:

Making homemade vegetable, chicken, or beef broth allows you to control the ingredients and reduce sodium. These broths can add depth to soups, stews, and sauces.

Additional Tips for Ingredient Substitutions, Cooking Methods, and Flavor Enhancement

Ingredient Substitutions

1. Spaghetti Squash for Pasta:

Roasted spaghetti squash can be a great low-calorie substitute for traditional pasta. It has a mild flavor that pairs well with a variety of sauces and toppings.

2. Chia Seeds for Eggs:

In baking, chia seeds mixed with water can replace eggs for a vegan and lower-calorie option. Mix one tablespoon of chia seeds with three tablespoons of water and let it sit for a few minutes to thicken.

3. Cottage Cheese for Ricotta Cheese:

Cottage cheese is lower in fat and calories compared to ricotta. It can be blended to a smooth consistency and used in lasagnas, stuffed shells, and desserts.

4. Plant-Based Milk for Dairy Milk:

Unsweetened almond, soy, or oat milk can replace dairy milk in recipes. These plant-based options are often lower in calories and can be chosen to suit dietary preferences.

5. Pureed Vegetables for Cream:

Pureed vegetables like carrots, sweet potatoes, or squash can add creaminess to soups and sauces without the added calories and fat of heavy cream.

6. Aquafaba for Egg Whites:

The liquid from canned chickpeas, known as aquafaba, can be whipped into a foam and used as a substitute for egg whites in meringues and baked goods.

Cooking Methods

Flavor Enhancement

1. Fermented Foods:

Adding fermented foods like kimchi, sauerkraut, and pickles to meals can provide a tangy, umami flavor. They also offer probiotics that are beneficial for gut health.

2. Infused Water:

Infusing water with fruits, herbs, and spices can create refreshing, flavored water that encourages hydration without added sugars. Try combinations like cucumber and mint, or berries and basil.

3. Roasting Nuts and Seeds:

Lightly roasting nuts and seeds enhances their flavor and crunch. Use them as toppings for salads, yogurt, or oatmeal for added texture and nutrition.

4. Using Umami-Rich Ingredients:

Ingredients like mushrooms, tomatoes, soy sauce, and nutritional yeast add umami, the savory fifth taste, which can make dishes more satisfying without adding extra calories.

5. Fresh Herbs:

Fresh herbs like basil, mint, and dill can add bright, fresh flavors to dishes. Adding them at the end of cooking or as a garnish ensures their flavors remain vibrant.

6. Citrus Marinades:

Marinating meats and vegetables in citrus juice (lemon, lime, or orange) can tenderize and flavor them without the need for high-calorie sauces.

7. Homemade Spice Blends:

Creating your own spice blends allows you to control the ingredients and avoid added sugars or preservatives found in store-bought versions. Experiment with blends like Italian seasoning, curry powder, or taco seasoning.

8. Smoked Paprika:

Adding smoked paprika to dishes can impart a rich, smoky flavor that mimics the taste of smoked meats or charred vegetables, enhancing the overall depth of flavor.

9. Using Broth Instead of Oil:

For sautéing and stir-frying, use a small amount of low-sodium vegetable or chicken broth instead of oil. This method adds moisture and flavor while reducing calories from fat.

10. Citrus Zests:

The zest of citrus fruits contains essential oils that provide a concentrated burst of flavor. Use a microplane to zest lemons, limes, or oranges over dishes to enhance their taste without extra calories.

11. Homemade Dressings and Sauces:

Making dressings and sauces at home allows you to control the ingredients and avoid added sugars and unhealthy fats. Use ingredients like Greek yogurt, mustard, vinegar, and fresh herbs for healthy and flavorful options.

By integrating these additional tips for ingredient substitutions, cooking methods, and flavor enhancement into my cooking routine, I've been able to create delicious, nutritious meals that support my weight management goals.

◆ ◆ ◆

RECIPE CATEGORIES

Breakfasts for Weight Loss

When it comes to breakfast, I've discovered that starting my day with a nutritious, balanced meal sets the tone for healthy eating throughout the day. Here are some of my favorite breakfasts that not only help with weight management but also keep me feeling full and energized.

High-Protein Smoothies

I love making smoothies because they're quick, versatile, and packed with nutrients. My go-to is a high-protein smoothie. I blend a scoop of protein powder with a handful of spinach, half a frozen banana, a tablespoon of chia seeds, and unsweetened almond milk. This combination provides protein, fiber, and healthy fats, keeping me satiated until lunch.

Overnight Oats

Overnight oats are a game-changer for busy mornings. The night before, I mix rolled oats with Greek yogurt, a splash of almond milk, and a teaspoon of honey. I then add chia seeds and a handful of berries. By morning, the oats are creamy and ready to eat. They're rich in fiber and protein, which helps control hunger and boost metabolism.

Veggie-Packed Omelet

Eggs are a fantastic source of protein, and I often make a veggie-packed omelet to kickstart my day. I sauté spinach, bell peppers, and onions in a non-stick pan, then add beaten eggs or egg whites. Sometimes, I sprinkle a little feta cheese on top for extra flavor. This breakfast is low in calories but high in nutrients, providing a satisfying start to my morning.

Avocado Toast with a Twist

Avocado toast is a classic, but I like to add my twist to make it more filling and nutritious. I mash half an avocado on whole-grain toast and top it with a poached egg. Sometimes, I add cherry tomatoes and a sprinkle of red pepper flakes for an extra kick. This meal is rich in healthy fats, fiber, and protein, keeping me full and satisfied.

Greek Yogurt Parfait

A Greek yogurt parfait is another quick and easy breakfast option. I layer Greek yogurt with fresh berries, a drizzle of honey, and a handful of granola. The yogurt provides protein, the berries add antioxidants and fiber, and the granola offers a satisfying crunch. It's a delicious and balanced breakfast that feels like a treat.

Chia Seed Pudding

Chia seed pudding is a favorite of mine for its convenience and health benefits. I mix chia seeds with unsweetened almond milk and a bit of vanilla extract, then let it sit overnight in the fridge. In the morning, I top it with sliced almonds and fresh fruit. Chia seeds are packed with fiber and omega-3 fatty acids, which help support weight loss and overall health.

Whole Grain Waffles with Fruit

When I have a bit more time, I make whole grain waffles using a mix of whole wheat flour and oats. I top them with Greek yogurt and fresh berries instead of syrup. This breakfast feels indulgent but is packed with fiber and protein, which helps keep blood sugar levels stable and reduces cravings throughout the day.

Smoothie Bowls

Smoothie bowls are a thicker version of smoothies that you can eat with a spoon. I blend frozen berries, a banana, spinach, and a bit of almond milk, then pour it into a bowl. I top it with granola, chia seeds, and sliced fruit. The combination of textures makes it satisfying, and it's a great way to pack in a variety of nutrients first thing in the morning.

Cottage Cheese with Fruit and Nuts

Cottage cheese is a protein powerhouse. I like to have it with a mix of fresh fruit like pineapple or berries and a sprinkle of nuts or seeds. This combination is low in calories but high in protein and healthy fats, keeping me full for hours.

Protein Pancakes

Protein pancakes are a great way to enjoy a classic breakfast while boosting protein intake. I make them by blending oats, cottage cheese, egg whites, and a scoop of protein powder. They cook up just like regular pancakes but offer a much higher protein content. I top them with fresh fruit and a bit of almond butter for a balanced meal.

These breakfast options have helped me stay on track with my weight loss goals while still enjoying delicious and satisfying meals. By focusing on protein, fiber, and healthy fats, I'm able to control hunger, maintain energy levels, and set a positive tone for the rest of the day.

◆ ◆ ◆

BREAKFASTS FOR WEIGHT LOSS: NUTRITIOUS AND SATISFYING RECIPES

When it comes to weight loss, starting the day with a nutritious and satisfying breakfast can make a big difference. Here are some of my favorite breakfast recipes that are both delicious and support weight loss goals.

1. High-Protein Berry Smoothie

Ingredients:

- ➤ 1 scoop of protein powder (vanilla or berry-flavored)
- ➤ 1 handful of spinach
- ➤ 1/2 frozen banana
- ➤ 1 cup of mixed berries (strawberries, blueberries, raspberries)
- ➤ 1 tablespoon of chia seeds
- ➤ 1 cup of unsweetened almond milk

Instructions:

- Combine all ingredients in a blender.
- Blend until smooth.
- Pour into a glass and enjoy immediately.

2. Overnight Oats

Ingredients:

- ➤ 1/2 cup of rolled oats
- ➤ 1/2 cup of Greek yogurt
- ➤ 1/2 cup of unsweetened almond milk
- ➤ 1 teaspoon of honey or maple syrup
- ➤ 1 tablespoon of chia seeds
- ➤ 1/2 cup of fresh berries

Instructions:

- In a mason jar or bowl, mix oats, Greek yogurt, almond milk, honey, and chia seeds.
- Stir well and cover. Refrigerate overnight.
- In the morning, top with fresh berries before eating.

3. Veggie-Packed Omelet

Ingredients:

➢ 2 eggs or 4 egg whites
➢ 1/2 cup of spinach, chopped
➢ 1/4 cup of bell peppers, diced
➢ 1/4 cup of onions, diced
➢ 1/4 cup of mushrooms, sliced
➢ Salt and pepper to taste
➢ 1 teaspoon of olive oil

Instructions:

- Heat olive oil in a non-stick pan over medium heat.
- Add onions, bell peppers, and mushrooms. Sauté until soft.
- Add spinach and cook until wilted.
- Beat eggs in a bowl and pour over the veggies in the pan.
- Cook until eggs are set, then fold the omelet in half.
- Season with salt and pepper, and serve hot.

4. Avocado Toast with a Poached Egg

Ingredients:

➢ 1 slice of whole-grain bread
➢ 1/2 ripe avocado
➢ 1 egg
➢ 1/4 cup of cherry tomatoes, halved
➢ Salt, pepper, and red pepper flakes to taste
➢ 1 teaspoon of lemon juice

Instructions:

- Toast the whole-grain bread until golden brown.
- Mash the avocado in a bowl and mix in lemon juice, salt, and pepper.
- Spread the avocado mixture on the toast.
- Poach the egg in simmering water until the white is set and the yolk is runny.
- Place the poached egg on top of the avocado toast.
- Top with cherry tomatoes and sprinkle with red pepper flakes.

5. Greek Yogurt Parfait

Ingredients:

- ➢ 1 cup of Greek yogurt
- ➢ 1/2 cup of fresh berries
- ➢ 1 tablespoon of honey
- ➢ 1/4 cup of granola

Instructions:

- In a glass or bowl, layer half of the Greek yogurt.
- Add half of the berries and drizzle with honey.
- Add the remaining Greek yogurt on top.
- Finish with the rest of the berries and a sprinkle of granola.

6. Chia Seed Pudding

Ingredients:

- ➢ 1/4 cup of chia seeds
- ➢ 1 cup of unsweetened almond milk
- ➢ 1 teaspoon of vanilla extract
- ➢ 1 tablespoon of honey or maple syrup
- ➢ Fresh fruit and nuts for topping

Instructions:

- In a bowl, mix chia seeds, almond milk, vanilla extract, and honey.
- Stir well to combine.
- Cover and refrigerate overnight.
- In the morning, stir the pudding and top with fresh fruit and nuts.

7. Whole Grain Waffles with Greek Yogurt and Berries

Ingredients:

- ➢ 1 cup of whole wheat flour
- ➢ 1/2 cup of oats
- ➢ 1 tablespoon of baking powder
- ➢ 1/4 teaspoon of salt
- ➢ 1 egg
- ➢ 1 cup of unsweetened almond milk
- ➢ 1/4 cup of Greek yogurt
- ➢ 1/2 cup of fresh berries

Instructions:

- Preheat your waffle maker.
- In a large bowl, mix flour, oats, baking powder, and salt.
- In another bowl, beat the egg and mix in almond milk.
- Combine the wet ingredients with the dry ingredients and stir until smooth.
- Pour the batter into the waffle maker and cook according to the manufacturer's instructions.
- Serve waffles topped with a dollop of Greek yogurt and fresh berries.

8. Smoothie Bowl

Ingredients:

- ➢ 1 frozen banana
- ➢ 1/2 cup of frozen berries
- ➢ 1/2 cup of spinach
- ➢ 1/2 cup of unsweetened almond milk
- ➢ 1/4 cup of granola
- ➢ Fresh fruit and chia seeds for topping

Instructions:

- In a blender, combine frozen banana, frozen berries, spinach, and almond milk.
- Blend until thick and smooth.
- Pour the smoothie into a bowl.
- Top with granola, fresh fruit, and chia seeds.

9. Cottage Cheese with Fruit and Nuts

Ingredients:

- ➢ 1 cup of cottage cheese
- ➢ 1/2 cup of pineapple chunks or fresh berries
- ➢ 2 tablespoons of chopped nuts (almonds, walnuts, or pecans)

Instructions:

- Spoon cottage cheese into a bowl.
- Top with pineapple chunks or berries.
- Sprinkle with chopped nuts.

10. Protein Pancakes

Ingredients:

- ➢ 1/2 cup of oats
- ➢ 1/2 cup of cottage cheese
- ➢ 1/2 cup of egg whites

- ➤ 1 scoop of protein powder (optional)
- ➤ 1/2 teaspoon of baking powder
- ➤ Fresh fruit and almond butter for topping

Instructions:

- Blend oats, cottage cheese, egg whites, protein powder, and baking powder until smooth.
- Heat a non-stick pan over medium heat and lightly coat with cooking spray.
- Pour batter into the pan to form pancakes.
- Cook until bubbles form on the surface, then flip and cook until golden brown.
- Serve with fresh fruit and a drizzle of almond butter.

11. Egg Muffins with Spinach and Feta

Ingredients:

- ➤ 6 eggs
- ➤ 1 cup of spinach, chopped
- ➤ 1/4 cup of feta cheese, crumbled
- ➤ Salt and pepper to taste
- ➤ Cooking spray

Instructions:

- Preheat the oven to 350°F (175°C). Grease a muffin tin with cooking spray.
- In a mixing bowl, whisk together the eggs until well beaten.
- Stir in chopped spinach, crumbled feta cheese, salt, and pepper.
- Pour the egg mixture evenly into the prepared muffin tin, filling each cup about three-quarters full.
- Bake in the preheated oven for 20-25 minutes, or until the egg muffins are set and slightly golden on top.
- 6. Allow the egg muffins to cool slightly before removing them from the muffin tin. Serve warm or refrigerate for later use.

12. Quinoa Breakfast Bowl

Ingredients:

- ➤ 1/2 cup of cooked quinoa
- ➤ 1/4 cup of Greek yogurt
- ➤ 1 tablespoon of honey
- ➤ 1/4 cup of mixed nuts and seeds (almonds, walnuts, sunflower seeds)
- ➤ 1/4 cup of fresh berries (strawberries, blueberries, raspberries)
- ➤ Dash of cinnamon (optional)

Instructions:

- In a bowl, layer cooked quinoa, Greek yogurt, and fresh berries.
- Drizzle honey over the top and sprinkle with mixed nuts and seeds.
- Add a dash of cinnamon for extra flavor, if desired.
- Mix everything together and enjoy!

13. Smoked Salmon Breakfast Wrap

Ingredients:

- ➢ 1 whole grain or low-carb tortilla
- ➢ 2 tablespoons of cream cheese
- ➢ 2 slices of smoked salmon
- ➢ 1/4 cup of cucumber, thinly sliced
- ➢ 1 tablespoon of capers
- ➢ Fresh dill for garnish

Instructions:

- Spread cream cheese evenly over the tortilla.
- Layer smoked salmon, cucumber slices, and capers on top of the cream cheese.
- Garnish with fresh dill.
- Roll up the tortilla into a wrap and slice in half. Serve immediately.

14. Tofu Scramble

Ingredients:

- ➢ 1/2 block of firm tofu, crumbled
- ➢ 1/4 cup of bell peppers, diced
- ➢ 1/4 cup of onions, diced
- ➢ 1/4 cup of cherry tomatoes, halved
- ➢ 1/4 teaspoon of turmeric
- ➢ Salt and pepper to taste
- ➢ 1 teaspoon of olive oil

Instructions:

- Heat olive oil in a skillet over medium heat.
- Add onions and bell peppers. Sauté until softened.
- Add crumbled tofu, cherry tomatoes, turmeric, salt, and pepper.
- Cook until tofu is heated through and vegetables are tender.
- Serve hot with whole grain toast or avocado slices.

15. Peanut Butter Banana Smoothie Bowl

Ingredients:

- ➤ 1 ripe banana, frozen
- ➤ 2 tablespoons of peanut butter
- ➤ 1/2 cup of unsweetened almond milk
- ➤ 1 tablespoon of chia seeds
- ➤ Toppings: sliced banana, granola, shredded coconut

Instructions:

- In a blender, combine frozen banana, peanut butter, almond milk, and chia seeds.
- Blend until smooth and creamy.
- Pour the smoothie into a bowl.
- Top with sliced banana, granola, and shredded coconut.
- Enjoy with a spoon!

These breakfast recipes are not only delicious but also designed to help you meet your weight loss goals.

◆ ◆ ◆

CONVENIENT AND NUTRITIOUS LUNCH RECIPES

Lunchtime is an opportunity to refuel your body with nutrients and energy for the rest of the day. These lunch recipes are not only convenient and delicious but also packed with nutrients to keep you satisfied and energized.

1. Quinoa Salad with Chickpeas and Roasted Vegetables

Ingredients:

- ➤ 1 cup quinoa, cooked
- ➤ 1 can chickpeas, rinsed and drained
- ➤ Assorted vegetables (bell peppers, zucchini, cherry tomatoes)
- ➤ Olive oil
- ➤ Salt and pepper
- ➤ Lemon vinaigrette (lemon juice, olive oil, minced garlic, honey)

Instructions:

- Preheat the oven to 400°F (200°C).
- Toss assorted vegetables with olive oil, salt, and pepper, then spread them on a baking sheet.
- Roast in the oven for 20-25 minutes until tender and slightly caramelized.
- In a large bowl, combine cooked quinoa, chickpeas, and roasted vegetables.
- Drizzle with lemon vinaigrette and toss to combine.
- Serve warm or cold.

2. Turkey and Hummus Wrap

Ingredients:

- ➤ Whole grain wrap
- ➤ Sliced turkey breast
- ➤ Hummus
- ➤ Baby spinach leaves
- ➤ Sliced cucumber
- ➤ Sliced tomato

Instructions:

- Lay the whole grain wrap flat on a clean surface.
- Spread a layer of hummus over the wrap.
- Layer sliced turkey breast, baby spinach leaves, sliced cucumber, and sliced tomato on top.
- Roll up the wrap tightly, folding in the sides as you go.
- Slice in half diagonally and serve.

3. Asian-Inspired Chicken Salad

Ingredients:

- Grilled chicken breast, sliced
- Mixed greens (spinach, arugula, lettuce)
- Shredded carrots
- Sliced bell peppers
- Edamame
- Sesame seeds
- Asian ginger dressing (soy sauce, rice vinegar, sesame oil, honey, minced ginger, minced garlic)

Instructions:

- In a large bowl, combine mixed greens, shredded carrots, sliced bell peppers, and edamame.
- Top with grilled chicken breast slices and sprinkle with sesame seeds.
- Drizzle with Asian ginger dressing and toss to coat.
- Serve immediately.

4. Veggie and Hummus Sandwich

Ingredients:

- Whole grain bread slices
- Hummus
- Sliced cucumber
- Sliced tomato
- Avocado slices
- Baby spinach leaves
- Sprouts (optional)

Instructions:

- Spread hummus on one side of each bread slice.
- Layer sliced cucumber, sliced tomato, avocado slices, baby spinach leaves, and sprouts on one bread slice.
- Top with the other bread slice to form a sandwich.
- Cut in half and serve.

5. Mediterranean Tuna Salad

Ingredients:

➢ Canned tuna, drained
➢ Diced cucumber
➢ Diced tomato
➢ Sliced red onion
➢ Kalamata olives, pitted and halved
➢ Crumbled feta cheese
➢ Fresh parsley, chopped
➢ Lemon juice
➢ Extra virgin olive oil
➢ Salt and pepper

Instructions:

- In a bowl, combine canned tuna, diced cucumber, diced tomato, sliced red onion, Kalamata olives, crumbled feta cheese, and chopped fresh parsley.
- Drizzle with lemon juice and extra virgin olive oil.
- Season with salt and pepper to taste.
- Toss gently to combine.
- Serve chilled.

6. Veggie and Bean Burrito Bowl

Ingredients:

➢ Cooked brown rice
➢ Black beans, rinsed and drained
➢ Sautéed bell peppers and onions
➢ Sliced avocado
➢ Salsa
➢ Greek yogurt or sour cream (optional)
➢ Fresh cilantro, chopped

Instructions:

- In a bowl, layer cooked brown rice, black beans, sautéed bell peppers and onions, sliced avocado, and salsa.
- Add a dollop of Greek yogurt or sour cream if desired.
- 3. Sprinkle with chopped fresh cilantro.
- 4. Serve as a burrito bowl or wrap in a tortilla for a convenient lunch option.

7. Chicken and Vegetable Stir-Fry

Ingredients:

- ➢ Sliced chicken breast
- ➢ Assorted vegetables (broccoli, bell peppers, snap peas, carrots)
- ➢ Garlic, minced
- ➢ Ginger, grated
- ➢ Soy sauce
- ➢ Sesame oil
- ➢ Cooked brown rice or quinoa

Instructions:

- Heat sesame oil in a skillet over medium-high heat.
- Add minced garlic and grated ginger, and stir-fry for a minute until fragrant.
- Add sliced chicken breast and cook until browned and cooked through.
- Add assorted vegetables and stir-fry until tender-crisp.
- Drizzle with soy sauce and toss to coat evenly.
- Serve over cooked brown rice or quinoa for a complete meal option.

8. Lentil and Vegetable Soup

Ingredients:

- ➢ Green or brown lentils
- ➢ Vegetable broth
- ➢ Onion, diced
- ➢ Carrots, diced
- ➢ Celery, diced
- ➢ Garlic, minced
- ➢ Cumin, paprika, and coriander (to taste)
- ➢ Fresh lemon juice
- ➢ Fresh parsley, chopped

Instructions:

- In a large pot, sauté diced onion, carrots, celery, and minced garlic until softened.
- Add green or brown lentils and vegetable broth to the pot.
- Season with cumin, paprika, and coriander to taste.
- Simmer the soup for 20-25 minutes, or until the lentils are tender.
- Stir in fresh lemon juice and chopped parsley before serving.
- Enjoy a hearty and flavorful vegetarian soup that's packed with protein and fiber.

9. Caprese Salad with Grilled Chicken

Ingredients:

- ➤ Grilled chicken breast, sliced
- ➤ Fresh mozzarella cheese, sliced
- ➤ Ripe tomatoes, sliced
- ➤ Fresh basil leaves
- ➤ Balsamic glaze
- ➤ Extra virgin olive oil
- ➤ Salt and pepper

Instructions:

- Arrange sliced tomatoes, fresh mozzarella cheese, and grilled chicken breast slices on a serving platter.
- Top with fresh basil leaves.
- Drizzle with balsamic glaze and extra virgin olive oil.
- Season with salt and pepper to taste.
- Serve as a light and refreshing salad option.

10. Veggie and Quinoa Stuffed Bell Peppers

Ingredients:

- ➤ Bell peppers, halved and seeds removed
- ➤ Cooked quinoa
- ➤ Black beans, rinsed and drained
- ➤ Corn kernels
- ➤ Diced tomatoes
- ➤ Diced red onion
- ➤ Chopped cilantro
- ➤ Ground cumin, chili powder, and garlic powder (to taste)
- ➤ Shredded cheese (optional)

Instructions:

- Preheat the oven to 375°F (190°C).
- In a large bowl, mix cooked quinoa, black beans, corn kernels, diced tomatoes, diced red onion, chopped cilantro, and seasonings.
- Stuff the halved bell peppers with the quinoa mixture.
- Place the stuffed peppers in a baking dish and cover with foil.
- Bake for 25-30 minutes until the peppers are tender.
- If desired, sprinkle shredded cheese on top during the last few minutes of baking.
- 7. Serve hot and enjoy!

These lunch recipes offer a variety of flavors and nutrients to keep you satisfied and energized throughout the day. Feel free to customize them based on your preferences and dietary needs.

WHOLESOME DINNER RECIPES FOR HEALTHY EATING

Dinner is an important meal that allows you to unwind and refuel after a long day. These dinner recipes are not only satisfying but also packed with nutrients to support your overall health and well-being.

1. Baked Salmon with Roasted Vegetables

Ingredients:

- ➢ Salmon fillets
- ➢ Assorted vegetables (such as broccoli, carrots, bell peppers)
- ➢ Olive oil
- ➢ Lemon slices
- ➢ Garlic powder, salt, and pepper

Instructions:

- Preheat the oven to 400°F (200°C).
- Place salmon fillets on a baking sheet lined with parchment paper.
- Season salmon with garlic powder, salt, and pepper. Top each fillet with a slice of lemon.
- Toss assorted vegetables with olive oil, salt, and pepper, then spread them on another baking sheet.
- Roast both the salmon and vegetables in the oven for 15-20 minutes, or until salmon is cooked through and vegetables are tender.
- Serve salmon with roasted vegetables for a nutritious and delicious dinner.

2. Quinoa Stuffed Bell Peppers

Ingredients:

- ➢ Bell peppers
- ➢ Cooked quinoa
- ➢ Black beans
- ➢ Corn kernels
- ➢ Diced tomatoes
- ➢ Diced red onion
- ➢ Chopped cilantro

- ➤ Ground cumin, chili powder, and garlic powder
- ➤ Shredded cheese (optional)

Instructions:

- Preheat the oven to 375°F (190°C).
- Cut the tops off bell peppers and remove seeds and membranes.
- In a large bowl, mix cooked quinoa, black beans, corn kernels, diced tomatoes, diced red onion, chopped cilantro, and seasonings.
- Stuff the bell peppers with the quinoa mixture.
- If desired, sprinkle shredded cheese on top of each stuffed pepper.
- Place stuffed peppers in a baking dish, cover with foil, and bake for 25-30 minutes.
- Remove foil and bake for an additional 5-10 minutes until cheese is melted and bubbly.
- Serve hot and enjoy a nutritious dinner.

3. Grilled Chicken and Vegetable Skewers

Ingredients:

- ➤ Chicken breast, cut into cubes
- ➤ Assorted vegetables (such as bell peppers, zucchini, cherry tomatoes)
- ➤ Olive oil
- ➤ Lemon juice
- ➤ Garlic, minced
- ➤ Italian seasoning
- ➤ Salt and pepper

Instructions:

- Preheat the grill to medium-high heat.
- In a bowl, combine chicken cubes with olive oil, lemon juice, minced garlic, Italian seasoning, salt, and pepper. Mix well to coat.
- Thread marinated chicken cubes and assorted vegetables onto skewers.
- Grill skewers for 10-15 minutes, turning occasionally, until chicken is cooked through and vegetables are tender.
- Serve hot and enjoy a flavorful and protein-rich dinner.

4. Vegetable Stir-Fry with Tofu

Ingredients:

- ➤ Firm tofu, cubed
- ➤ Assorted vegetables (such as broccoli, snap peas, bell peppers, carrots)
- ➤ Garlic, minced
- ➤ Ginger, grated
- ➤ Soy sauce

- ➤ Sesame oil
- ➤ Cooked brown rice or quinoa

Instructions:

- Heat sesame oil in a large skillet or wok over medium-high heat.
- Add minced garlic and grated ginger, and stir-fry for a minute until fragrant.
- Add cubed tofu and cook until lightly browned on all sides.
- Add assorted vegetables and stir-fry until tender-crisp.
- Drizzle with soy sauce and toss to coat evenly.
- Serve vegetable stir-fry over cooked brown rice or quinoa for a wholesome and satisfying dinner.

5. Lentil and Vegetable Soup

Ingredients:

- ➤ Green or brown lentils
- ➤ Vegetable broth
- ➤ Onion, diced
- ➤ Carrots, diced
- ➤ Celery, diced
- ➤ Garlic, minced
- ➤ Cumin, paprika, and coriander
- ➤ Fresh lemon juice
- ➤ Fresh parsley, chopped

Instructions:

- In a large pot, sauté diced onion, carrots, celery, and minced garlic until softened.
- Add green or brown lentils and vegetable broth to the pot.
- Season with cumin, paprika, and coriander to taste.
- Simmer the soup for 20-25 minutes, or until the lentils are tender.
- Stir in fresh lemon juice and chopped parsley before serving.
- 6. Enjoy a hearty and nutritious lentil soup for dinner.

6. Veggie and Chickpea Curry

Ingredients:

- ➤ Chickpeas, cooked
- ➤ Assorted vegetables (such as cauliflower, bell peppers, peas)
- ➤ Onion, diced
- ➤ Garlic, minced
- ➤ Ginger, grated
- ➤ Curry powder, turmeric, and cumin

- ➤ Coconut milk
- ➤ Fresh cilantro, chopped
- ➤ Cooked rice or naan bread

Instructions:

- In a large skillet, sauté diced onion, minced garlic, and grated ginger until softened.
- Add assorted vegetables and cook until slightly tender.
- Stir in cooked chickpeas and season with curry powder, turmeric, and cumin.
- Pour in coconut milk and simmer for 10-15 minutes.
- Garnish with chopped fresh cilantro before serving.
- Serve veggie and chickpea curry over cooked rice or with naan bread for a flavorful dinner option.

7. Spaghetti Squash with Marinara Sauce

Ingredients:

- ➤ Spaghetti squash
- ➤ Marinara sauce
- ➤ Fresh basil leaves
- ➤ Grated Parmesan cheese (optional)

Instructions:

- Preheat the oven to 375°F (190°C).
- Cut the spaghetti squash in half lengthwise and scoop out the seeds.
- Place the squash halves, cut side down, on a baking sheet lined with parchment paper.
- 4. Bake for 40-45 minutes, or until the squash is tender and easily pierced with a fork.
- 5. Use a fork to scrape the flesh of the squash into strands.
- 6. Heat marinara sauce in a saucepan and pour over the spaghetti squash.
- 7. Garnish with fresh basil leaves and grated Parmesan cheese if desired.
- 8. Serve hot and enjoy a low-carb and nutritious dinner.

These dinner recipes offer a variety of flavors and ingredients to keep your meals exciting while supporting your health. Feel free to customize them based on your preferences and dietary needs.

HEALTHY SNACK OPTIONS AND GUILT-FREE TREATS

Snacking can be a great way to keep your energy levels up throughout the day, but it's important to choose options that are both satisfying and nutritious. Here are some healthy snack ideas and treats that allow for smart indulgence without derailing your progress:

1. Greek Yogurt with Berries

Ingredients:

> Greek yogurt
> Mixed berries (such as strawberries, blueberries, raspberries)
> Honey (optional)

Instructions:

- Spoon Greek yogurt into a bowl or serving cup.
- Top with mixed berries.
- Drizzle with honey for added sweetness if desired.
- Enjoy a creamy and satisfying snack packed with protein and antioxidants.

2. Homemade Trail Mix

Ingredients:

> Raw almonds
> Walnuts
> Cashews
> Pumpkin seeds
> Dried cranberries or raisins
> Dark chocolate chips or chunks

Instructions:

- Mix together raw almonds, walnuts, cashews, pumpkin seeds, dried cranberries or raisins, and dark chocolate chips or chunks in a bowl.
- Portion out into small bags or containers for convenient snacking on the go.
- Enjoy a nutrient-rich and satisfying trail mix that provides a balance of healthy fats, protein, and carbohydrates.

3. Apple Slices with Peanut Butter

Ingredients:

- ➢ Apple, sliced
- ➢ Peanut butter (or almond butter for a variation)

Instructions:

- Spread peanut butter on apple slices.
- Enjoy the crunchy texture of the apple paired with the creamy nut butter for a satisfying and nutritious snack.
- Optionally, sprinkle with cinnamon or drizzle with honey for added flavor.

4. Veggie Sticks with Hummus

Ingredients:

- ➢ Assorted vegetable sticks (such as carrots, celery, bell peppers, cucumber)
- ➢ Hummus

Instructions:

- Cut assorted vegetables into sticks or slices.
- Serve with a side of hummus for dipping.
- Enjoy a crunchy and refreshing snack packed with fiber, vitamins, and minerals.

5. Rice Cake with Avocado and Cherry Tomatoes

Ingredients:

- ➢ Rice cake
- ➢ Avocado, mashed
- ➢ Cherry tomatoes, halved
- ➢ Salt and pepper

Instructions:

- Spread mashed avocado on a rice cake.
- Top with halved cherry tomatoes.
- Season with salt and pepper to taste.
- Enjoy a light and satisfying snack that combines creamy avocado with juicy tomatoes.

6. Cottage Cheese with Pineapple

Ingredients:

- ➢ Cottage cheese
- ➢ Fresh pineapple chunks

Instructions:

- Spoon cottage cheese into a bowl.
- Top with fresh pineapple chunks.
- Enjoy a creamy and tropical snack that's rich in protein and vitamin C.

7. Dark Chocolate Covered Almonds

Ingredients:

- ➢ Raw almonds
- ➢ Dark chocolate (at least 70% cocoa)

Instructions:

- Melt dark chocolate in a double boiler or microwave.
- Dip raw almonds into the melted chocolate to coat.
- Place chocolate-covered almonds on a parchment-lined baking sheet.
- Allow chocolate to set at room temperature or in the refrigerator.
- Enjoy a sweet and satisfying treat that provides a combination of antioxidants and healthy fats.

8. Frozen Yogurt Bark

Ingredients:

- ➢ Greek yogurt
- ➢ Honey or maple syrup
- ➢ Fresh fruit (such as berries, sliced bananas, kiwi)
- ➢ Granola or chopped nuts

Instructions:

- Mix Greek yogurt with honey or maple syrup to sweeten.
- Spread the sweetened yogurt onto a parchment-lined baking sheet.
- Top with fresh fruit and granola or chopped nuts.
- Freeze until firm, then break into pieces.
- Enjoy a refreshing and customizable frozen treat that's perfect for satisfying cravings.

9. Air-Popped Popcorn with Sea Salt

Ingredients:

- ➢ Popcorn kernels

➢ Sea salt

Instructions:

- Air-pop popcorn kernels according to package instructions.
- Sprinkle with sea salt to taste.
- Enjoy a light and crunchy snack that's low in calories and high in fiber.

10. Frozen Grapes

Ingredients:

➢ Grapes

Instructions:

- Wash grapes and remove stems.
- Place grapes in a single layer on a baking sheet.
- Freeze until firm.
- Enjoy a refreshing and naturally sweet snack that's perfect for hot days.

These healthy snack options and guilt-free treats provide delicious ways to satisfy cravings while supporting your overall health and wellness goals. Feel free to mix and match ingredients to create your own favorite combinations.

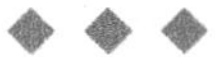

MEAL PLANNING AND PREPARATION

C omes to meal planning and preparation for weight loss, I've found a few key strategies that really make a difference:

➤ Know Your Goals: First things first, it's important to have a clear idea of what you want to achieve. Whether it's shedding a few pounds or simply eating healthier, knowing your goals will help guide your meal planning decisions.

➤ Start with the Basics: Begin by taking stock of what you already have in your kitchen. Then, think about the meals you enjoy and the foods that make you feel good. From there, you can start to build your meal plan.

➤ Keep it Balanced: When planning your meals, aim for a balance of protein, healthy fats, complex carbohydrates, and plenty of fruits and veggies. This will help keep you feeling satisfied and energized throughout the day.

➤ Prep Ahead: One of the biggest game-changers for me has been prepping ingredients ahead of time. Spend a little time on the weekend washing and chopping veggies, cooking grains and proteins, and portioning out snacks. This makes it so much easier to throw together a healthy meal during the week when things get busy.

➤ Get Creative: Don't be afraid to experiment with new recipes and flavors. This can help keep things interesting and prevent mealtime boredom.

➤ Listen to Your Body: Pay attention to your hunger and fullness cues, and eat mindfully. This can help prevent overeating and promote a healthy relationship with food.

➤ Stay Flexible: While it's important to stick to your meal plan as much as possible, it's also okay to be flexible. Life happens, and sometimes you might need to make adjustments on the fly. Just do your best to make healthy choices whenever you can.

➤ Track Your Progress: Keep track of your meals and how they make you feel. This can help you identify patterns and make adjustments as needed.

➢ Stay Positive: Finally, remember that weight loss is a journey, and it's okay to have ups and downs along the way. Stay positive, stay focused on your goals, and celebrate your progress, no matter how small.

These tips and staying consistent with your meal planning and preparation, you can set yourself up for success on your weight loss journey. Trust me, it's worth the effort!

Here are some tips based on my personal experience to make healthy eating more accessible and convenient through grocery shopping, batch cooking, and meal prepping:

Grocery Shopping Tips

➢ Plan Ahead: Take some time to plan your meals for the week before heading to the grocery store. This will help you create a list of the ingredients you need and avoid wandering aimlessly through the aisles.

➢ Stick to the Perimeter: Focus on shopping the perimeter of the store where you'll find fresh produce, lean proteins, and dairy products. This is where the majority of whole, nutrient-dense foods are located.

➢ Read Labels: When purchasing packaged foods, take a moment to read the nutrition labels. Look for products with minimal ingredients, low added sugars, and minimal processing.

➢ Buy in Bulk: Consider buying staple items like grains, beans, and nuts in bulk to save money and reduce waste. Just make sure you have enough storage space at home.

➢ Choose Seasonal Produce: Opt for fruits and vegetables that are in season, as they tend to be fresher, more flavorful, and more affordable. Plus, you'll be supporting local farmers.

Batch Cooking Tips

➢ Schedule Time for Batch Cooking: Set aside a few hours on the weekend or whenever works best for your schedule to batch cook your meals for the week. This will save you time and energy during busy weekdays.

➢ Keep it Simple: Choose a few staple recipes that you enjoy and that can be easily batch cooked in large quantities. This could be soups, stews, casseroles, or roasted vegetables.

➢ Invest in Quality Storage Containers: Invest in a set of quality storage containers that are microwave-safe, dishwasher-safe, and free of harmful chemicals. Glass containers are durable and ideal for storing batch-cooked meals.

➤ Label and Date: Once your meals are cooked and portioned out, be sure to label them with the contents and date. This will help you keep track of what's in your fridge and ensure nothing goes to waste.

➤ Freeze Portions: If you've batch cooked more than you can eat in a week, portion out the extras and freeze them for later. This way, you'll always have healthy meals on hand when you need them.

Meal Prepping Tips

➤ Prep Ingredients Ahead of Time: Wash and chop fruits and vegetables, cook grains and proteins, and portion out snacks ahead of time. This will make it easier to assemble meals during the week.

➤ Mix and Match Ingredients: Prepare versatile ingredients that can be mixed and matched to create different meals throughout the week. For example, cook a batch of quinoa that can be used in salads, stir-fries, or grain bowls.

➤ Use Time-Saving Appliances: Take advantage of time-saving appliances like a slow cooker, Instant Pot, or air fryer to streamline the meal prep process. These appliances can help you cook large batches of food with minimal effort.

➤ Portion Out Meals: Once your meals are prepped, portion them out into individual containers for easy grab-and-go lunches and dinners. This will help you stay on track with your healthy eating goals, even when you're short on time.

➤ Stay Organized: Keep your fridge and pantry organized so you can easily see what ingredients you have on hand and avoid letting anything go to waste.

By incorporating these tips into your grocery shopping, batch cooking, and meal prepping routine, you can make healthy eating more accessible and convenient in your day-to-day life. With a little planning and preparation, you'll be well-equipped to stick to your healthy eating goals and enjoy nutritious meals throughout the week.

◆ ◆ ◆

PHYSICAL ACTIVITY AND LIFESTYLE FACTORS

From a personal perspective, I can't emphasize enough the importance of physical activity in conjunction with healthy eating for sustainable weight management. Here's why:

➤ Burns Calories: Engaging in physical activity helps you burn calories, which is essential for creating a calorie deficit and losing weight. When combined with a balanced diet, exercise can accelerate weight loss and improve overall body composition.

➤ Boosts Metabolism: Regular exercise can boost your metabolism, helping your body burn calories more efficiently even when you're at rest. This can make it easier to maintain a healthy weight over the long term.

➤ Preserves Lean Muscle Mass: When you lose weight, you want to ensure that you're losing fat mass rather than muscle mass. Incorporating strength training into your exercise routine helps preserve lean muscle mass, which is important for maintaining metabolic health and preventing weight regain.

➤ Improves Mood and Energy Levels: Exercise releases endorphins, which are feel-good hormones that can improve your mood and reduce stress and anxiety. Additionally, regular physical activity can increase energy levels and improve overall mental well-being, making it easier to stay motivated and committed to your weight loss journey.

➤ Supports Overall Health: In addition to its benefits for weight management, regular physical activity is essential for overall health and well-being. It can reduce the risk of chronic diseases such as heart disease, diabetes, and certain cancers, and improve cardiovascular health, bone density, and immune function.

➤ Enhances Quality of Life: Being active allows you to participate in daily activities with greater ease and enjoyment. Whether it's going for a hike, playing with your kids, or simply taking a leisurely stroll, physical activity enhances your quality of life and promotes longevity.

In summary, incorporating regular physical activity into your routine is essential for sustainable weight management and overall health. When combined with healthy eating habits, exercise can help you achieve and maintain a healthy weight, improve body composition, boost metabolism, enhance mood and energy levels, and support long-term well-being. So, lace up those sneakers, find activities you enjoy, and make physical activity a priority in your daily life. Your body will thank you for it!

Here are some practical tips for incorporating exercise into your daily routine and maintaining an active lifestyle:

- ➤ Set Realistic Goals: Start by setting realistic and achievable exercise goals based on your current fitness level and schedule. Whether it's going for a 30-minute walk every day or hitting the gym three times a week, setting specific goals will help you stay focused and motivated.

- ➤ Find Activities You Enjoy: Choose activities that you enjoy and look forward to doing. Whether it's swimming, dancing, cycling, hiking, or playing a sport, finding activities that you genuinely enjoy will make it easier to stick to your exercise routine.

- ➤ Schedule Exercise into Your Day: Treat exercise like any other appointment and schedule it into your day. Whether you prefer to exercise in the morning, during your lunch break, or in the evening, block off time in your calendar for physical activity and prioritize it just like you would any other commitment.

- ➤ Make it Convenient: Choose activities that are convenient and accessible based on your lifestyle and preferences. If you enjoy outdoor activities, explore nearby parks or trails. If you prefer working out at home, invest in some basic exercise equipment or follow online workout videos.

- ➤ Incorporate Exercise into Daily Activities: Look for opportunities to sneak in extra physical activity throughout your day. Take the stairs instead of the elevator, walk or bike to work if possible, park farther away from your destination, or do a quick workout during TV commercial breaks.

- ➤ Mix it Up: Keep your exercise routine varied and interesting by mixing up your activities. Incorporate a combination of cardiovascular exercise, strength training, flexibility, and balance exercises to keep your body challenged and prevent boredom.

- ➤ Find Accountability Partners: Enlist the support of friends, family members, or coworkers to help you stay accountable to your exercise goals. Whether it's joining a fitness class together, going for walks during lunch breaks, or simply checking in with each other regularly, having accountability partners can help keep you motivated and accountable.

- ➤ Track Your Progress: Keep track of your workouts, progress, and achievements to stay motivated and see how far you've come. Use a fitness app, journal, or calendar to track your workouts, set milestones, and celebrate your successes along the way.

➤ Listen to Your Body: Pay attention to your body's cues and adjust your exercise routine as needed. If you're feeling fatigued or experiencing pain, give yourself permission to take a rest day or modify your workouts accordingly. Remember that rest is an essential part of any exercise routine and allows your body to recover and repair.

➤ Be Flexible: Lastly, be flexible and adaptable with your exercise routine. Life can be unpredictable, and there will inevitably be days when things don't go as planned. Instead of getting discouraged, be flexible and find alternative ways to stay active, even if it's just a short walk or a few minutes of stretching.

By incorporating these practical tips into your daily routine, you can make exercise a natural and enjoyable part of your lifestyle. Remember that consistency is key, so find activities you love, set realistic goals, and make physical activity a priority in your daily life.

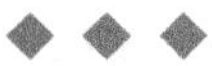

OVERCOMING CHALLENGES AND PLATEAUS

The common challenges and obstacles readers may encounter on their weight loss journey:

➤ Emotional Eating Battles: From personal experience, emotional eating has been a constant challenge. During stressful times or moments of boredom, turning to food for comfort feels like second nature. Breaking this cycle requires a deep dive into understanding the emotional triggers behind such behaviors and finding alternative coping mechanisms.

➤ Cravings and Temptations: Oh, the allure of cravings and temptations! Whether it's the aroma of freshly baked pastries or the sight of a favorite dessert, resisting temptation can feel like a Herculean task. Developing strategies to manage cravings, such as distraction techniques or indulging in healthier alternatives, has been key in navigating these moments.

➤ Social Situations and Peer Pressure: Social gatherings and outings often revolve around food, which can present a minefield of challenges. Whether it's resisting peer pressure to overeat or navigating restaurant menus with limited healthy options, maintaining willpower in social settings requires assertiveness and planning ahead.

➤ Self-Doubt and Negative Self-Talk: Wrestling with self-doubt and negative self-talk is an ongoing battle. There are days when doubts creep in, questioning whether the effort is worth it or if success is even achievable. Cultivating self-compassion and practicing positive affirmations have been instrumental in combating these inner demons.

➤ Time Constraints and Busy Schedules: Balancing the demands of work, family, and personal commitments while prioritizing exercise and meal prep is no small feat. Finding pockets of time amidst a busy schedule for workouts and healthy meal planning requires careful time management and flexibility.

➤ Weight Loss Plateaus: Ah, the dreaded plateau—a frustrating roadblock on the journey to weight loss. After initial progress, hitting a plateau can feel disheartening and demotivating. It's during these times that perseverance and patience are put to the test, with a focus on adjusting strategies and staying the course.

➤ Lack of Support or Understanding: Surrounding oneself with supportive individuals who understand the challenges of the weight loss journey is invaluable. However, not everyone may offer the encouragement or empathy needed. Seeking out like-minded communities, whether online or in-person, can provide the understanding and solidarity needed to stay motivated.

These challenges requires resilience, self-awareness, and a willingness to adapt. While the path may be fraught with obstacles, each hurdle overcome brings one step closer to achieving lasting success on the weight loss journey.

Some strategies for overcoming plateaus, staying motivated, and staying on track from a personal perspective:

➢ Mix Up Your Routine: Plateaus often occur when your body adapts to your current exercise and eating habits. Shake things up by trying new workouts, varying the intensity or duration of your exercises, or experimenting with different types of physical activity. Similarly, explore new healthy recipes and meal options to keep your taste buds excited and your body guessing.

➢ Set Small, Achievable Goals: Break your larger weight loss goal into smaller, more manageable milestones. Celebrating these mini victories along the way can provide a much-needed boost in motivation and keep you focused on your progress. Whether it's fitting into a smaller clothing size, increasing your workout endurance, or hitting a certain number on the scale, every achievement counts.

➢ Find Your Why: Reflect on the reasons behind your desire to lose weight and improve your health. Whether it's to feel more confident, improve your energy levels, or set a positive example for your loved ones, reconnecting with your underlying motivations can reignite your passion and determination during challenging times.

➢ Visualize Success: Create a mental image of what success looks and feels like to you. Whether it's envisioning yourself reaching your goal weight, crossing the finish line of a race, or simply feeling more confident and vibrant in your everyday life, visualization can help reinforce your commitment and keep you focused on the end goal.

➢ Practice Self-Compassion: Be kind to yourself during periods of struggle or setbacks. Weight loss journeys are rarely linear, and it's normal to encounter obstacles along the way. Instead of berating yourself for perceived failures, practice self-compassion and remind yourself that progress is made through persistence, not perfection.

➢ Seek Support and Accountability: Surround yourself with a supportive network of friends, family, or fellow weight loss enthusiasts who understand your journey and can offer encouragement and guidance. Whether it's joining a fitness class, participating in online communities, or enlisting a workout buddy, having accountability partners can help keep you motivated and accountable.

➤ Focus on Non-Scale Victories: While the number on the scale is one measure of progress, it's important to celebrate other indicators of success along the way. Pay attention to how your clothes fit, improvements in your energy levels and mood, increases in strength and stamina, and other non-scale victories that demonstrate your progress and hard work.

➤ Practice Patience and Persistence: Remember that sustainable weight loss takes time and consistent effort. Plateaus and setbacks are a natural part of the journey, but they don't define your ultimate success. Stay patient, stay persistent, and trust in the process, knowing that each day you're moving closer to your goals.

➤ Track Your Progress: Keep a journal or use a tracking app to record your workouts, meals, and progress towards your goals. Seeing how far you've come can be incredibly motivating and provide a tangible reminder of your achievements. Celebrate your successes, no matter how small, and use setbacks as learning opportunities rather than reasons to give up.

➤ Reward Yourself: Set up a system of rewards for reaching milestones or sticking to your healthy habits. Treat yourself to something special, like a massage, a new workout outfit, or a night out with friends, as a way to acknowledge your hard work and dedication. Just be sure to choose rewards that align with your health and fitness goals.

➤ Visual Cues: Surround yourself with visual reminders of your goals and aspirations. Create a vision board with images and quotes that inspire you, or place motivational notes and affirmations in prominent places where you'll see them daily. These visual cues can serve as constant reminders of why you're working towards your goals and help keep you focused and motivated.

➤ Find Joy in Movement: Instead of viewing exercise as a chore, find activities that bring you joy and fulfillment. Whether it's dancing, hiking in nature, practicing yoga, or playing a sport you love, incorporating activities that you genuinely enjoy into your routine can make exercise feel less like work and more like play.

➤ Practice Mindfulness: Incorporate mindfulness practices into your daily routine to help you stay present and focused on your goals. Whether it's mindful eating, meditation, or simply taking a few moments each day to breathe deeply and center yourself, mindfulness can help reduce stress, increase self-awareness, and improve overall well-being.

➤ Stay Flexible: Life is unpredictable, and there will inevitably be days when things don't go as planned. Instead of letting setbacks derail your progress, stay flexible and adapt to changing circumstances. If you miss a workout or indulge in an unplanned treat, don't dwell on it—simply acknowledge it, learn from it, and move on with renewed determination.

➤ Visualize Your Future Self: Take a moment to imagine yourself in the future, living your healthiest, happiest life. Visualize how you'll look, feel, and move with confidence and vitality. By keeping this vision of your future self in mind, you can stay motivated and inspired to continue making positive choices each day.

These strategies into your weight loss journey, you can overcome plateaus, stay motivated, and stay on track towards achieving your goals. Remember that progress may not always be linear, but with patience, perseverance, and a positive mindset, you can create lasting change and transform your life for the better.

◆ ◆ ◆

MAINTAINING LONG-TERM SUCCESS

Some strategies for maintaining weight loss results and adopting healthy habits for life:

➤ Find Your Why: Reflect on the reasons behind your desire to maintain weight loss and adopt healthy habits for life. Whether it's improving your overall health, setting a positive example for your loved ones, or simply feeling more confident and vibrant, reconnecting with your underlying motivations can reignite your passion and determination.

➤ Create a Supportive Environment: Surround yourself with people, places, and things that support your health and wellness goals. Seek out friends, family members, or online communities who share your values and can provide encouragement, accountability, and motivation. Similarly, create an environment at home and at work that makes it easier to make healthy choices, such as keeping nutritious foods on hand and making physical activity a regular part of your routine.

➤ Set Realistic Goals: Establish realistic and achievable goals that align with your long-term vision for health and well-being. Break larger goals into smaller, more manageable steps, and celebrate your progress along the way. Remember that sustainable change takes time, and focus on making gradual improvements rather than expecting overnight results.

➤ Practice Self-Compassion: Be kind to yourself throughout the process of maintaining weight loss and adopting healthy habits. Embrace imperfection and recognize that setbacks and challenges are a normal part of the journey. Instead of criticizing yourself for perceived failures, practice self-compassion and treat yourself with the same kindness and understanding that you would offer to a friend.

➤ Embrace Variety and Flexibility: Avoid falling into a rigid or restrictive mindset when it comes to diet and exercise. Instead, embrace variety and flexibility in your approach, allowing for different types of foods and activities that bring you joy and satisfaction. Find enjoyment in trying new recipes, exploring different forms of physical activity, and adapting your routine to fit your changing needs and preferences.

➤ Prioritize Self-Care: Make self-care a priority in your daily life, taking time to nourish your body, mind, and soul. This might include getting enough sleep, managing stress through relaxation techniques like meditation or yoga, spending time outdoors in nature, engaging in creative pursuits or hobbies, and nurturing your relationships with loved ones. By taking care of yourself holistically, you'll support your overall health and well-being and make it easier to maintain healthy habits for life.

➢ Practice Mindful Eating: Cultivate a mindful approach to eating, paying attention to your body's hunger and fullness cues, and savoring each bite of food. Avoid distractions like screens or multitasking while eating, and choose foods that nourish your body and satisfy your cravings in a balanced and satisfying way. By practicing mindful eating, you'll develop a healthier relationship with food and make more conscious choices that support your long-term health and wellness.

➢ Stay Active and Find Joy in Movement: Make physical activity a regular part of your routine, choosing activities that you enjoy and that fit into your lifestyle. Whether it's going for a walk, dancing, cycling, or practicing yoga, find activities that bring you joy and make you feel good. Focus on the benefits of movement beyond weight loss, such as improved mood, increased energy levels, and enhanced overall well-being.

➢ Celebrate Your Successes: Take time to celebrate your successes, no matter how small, and acknowledge the progress you've made on your journey. Whether it's reaching a milestone on the scale, mastering a new healthy recipe, or completing a challenging workout, celebrate your achievements and give yourself credit for your hard work and dedication. By celebrating your successes, you'll stay motivated and inspired to continue making positive changes in your life.

➢ Stay Curious and Keep Learning: Approach your health and wellness journey with a spirit of curiosity and openness, and be willing to explore new ideas, strategies, and approaches along the way. Stay informed about the latest research and developments in nutrition, fitness, and well-being, and be willing to adapt your approach based on new information and insights. By staying curious and keeping learning, you'll continue to grow and evolve on your journey towards lifelong health and happiness.

➢ Practice Gratitude: Cultivate an attitude of gratitude for your body and all that it allows you to do. Focus on the positive aspects of your health journey, such as increased energy, improved mood, and a greater sense of well-being. Take time each day to express gratitude for the progress you've made and the opportunity to live a healthy, fulfilling life.

➢ Stay Consistent, Not Perfect: Remember that consistency, not perfection, is key to long-term success. Aim for progress, not perfection, and focus on making sustainable changes that you can maintain over time. If you have a setback or slip-up, don't let it derail your progress. Instead, refocus on your goals and get back on track as soon as possible.

➢ Find Healthy Coping Mechanisms: Develop healthy coping mechanisms for dealing with stress, emotions, and challenges in life. Instead of turning to food for comfort, find alternative ways to manage stress and soothe your emotions, such as practicing deep breathing, journaling, spending time in nature, or talking to a trusted friend or therapist.

➤ Practice Self-Reflection: Take time to reflect on your health journey regularly and assess what's working well and what could be improved. Be honest with yourself about your habits and behaviors, and identify areas where you could make positive changes. Use self-reflection as an opportunity for growth and self-improvement.

➤ Stay Engaged and Inspired: Stay engaged and inspired on your health journey by seeking out sources of motivation and inspiration. Whether it's reading books and articles, listening to podcasts, following inspiring individuals on social media, or joining online communities, surround yourself with positivity and encouragement that uplifts and motivates you.

➤ Be Your Own Advocate: Take ownership of your health and well-being by advocating for yourself and your needs. Educate yourself about nutrition, fitness, and wellness, and be proactive in seeking out the resources and support you need to thrive. Trust your instincts and listen to your body, and don't be afraid to speak up and ask for help when you need it.

➤ Set Boundaries: Set boundaries to protect your health and well-being, both physically and emotionally. Learn to say no to things that don't align with your values or support your goals, whether it's unhealthy foods, negative influences, or stressful situations. Prioritize your health and make choices that honor your body and mind.

➤ Celebrate Every Step: Celebrate every step of your health journey, no matter how small. Whether it's making a healthy choice at a meal, completing a workout, or simply showing up for yourself each day, acknowledge and celebrate your efforts and accomplishments. Remember that every positive choice you make brings you closer to your goals.

➤ Practice Patience: Be patient with yourself and trust the process of change. Rome wasn't built in a day, and sustainable change takes time. Stay committed to your health goals, even when progress feels slow or obstacles arise. Trust that each step you take, no matter how small, is moving you in the right direction.

➤ Be Kind to Yourself: Above all, be kind to yourself throughout your health journey. Treat yourself with the same compassion, understanding, and respect that you would offer to a loved one. Celebrate your strengths, forgive your shortcomings, and embrace the journey with kindness and grace.

These strategies into your life, you can maintain your weight loss results and adopt healthy habits that support your overall health and well-being for years to come. Remember that your health journey is unique to you, and there's no one-size-fits-all approach. Find what works best for you and embrace the journey with openness, curiosity, and self-compassion.

Guidance on building a supportive environment and mindset for long-term success from a personal viewpoint:

> Surround Yourself with Positivity: Surround yourself with people, places, and things that uplift and inspire you. Seek out friends, family members, or online communities who share your health and wellness goals and can provide encouragement, support, and accountability. Surround yourself with positive influences that reinforce your commitment to living a healthy, vibrant life.

> Create a Healthy Living Space: Create an environment at home and at work that supports your health and wellness goals. Stock your kitchen with nutritious foods and ingredients, and make healthy eating easy and accessible by organizing your pantry, fridge, and meal prep areas. Similarly, create an inviting space for physical activity, whether it's setting up a home gym, designating a yoga corner, or simply keeping your workout gear easily accessible.

> Practice Daily Affirmations: Incorporate positive affirmations into your daily routine to cultivate a supportive mindset and reinforce your commitment to long-term success. Start each day with affirmations that resonate with you, such as "I am strong, healthy, and capable," "I trust in my ability to make healthy choices," or "I am worthy of investing in my health and well-being." Repeat these affirmations throughout the day to stay focused and motivated.

> Visualize Your Success: Take time each day to visualize your success and imagine yourself achieving your health and wellness goals. Close your eyes and picture yourself living your healthiest, happiest life, feeling vibrant, energized, and confident in your body. Visualize the specific actions you'll take to reach your goals and the positive outcomes that will result from your efforts. By visualizing your success, you'll stay motivated and inspired to take action each day.

> Practice Gratitude: Cultivate an attitude of gratitude for your body, your health, and all the blessings in your life. Take time each day to express gratitude for the progress you've made on your health journey, as well as the support and resources that have helped you along the way. Focus on the positive aspects of your life and health, and let gratitude guide your mindset and actions.

> Set Intentions: Set clear intentions for how you want to live your life and prioritize your health and well-being. Take time to reflect on your values, priorities, and goals, and identify the actions you can take to align your life with your intentions. Whether it's setting aside time for self-care, prioritizing movement and exercise, or nourishing your body with nutritious foods, set intentions that support your long-term health and happiness.

> Practice Self-Compassion: Be kind to yourself throughout your health journey and treat

yourself with the same compassion, understanding, and respect that you would offer to a loved one. Embrace imperfection and recognize that setbacks and challenges are a normal part of the journey. Instead of criticizing yourself for perceived failures, practice self-compassion and treat yourself with gentleness and grace.

➤ Stay Present: Stay present and mindful in each moment, focusing on the here and now rather than dwelling on the past or worrying about the future. Pay attention to your thoughts, feelings, and sensations without judgment, and savor the simple joys and pleasures of everyday life. By staying present, you'll cultivate a greater sense of peace, contentment, and fulfillment in your life.

➤ Embrace Change: Embrace change as a natural and inevitable part of life, and approach it with curiosity, openness, and resilience. Be willing to adapt to new circumstances, explore new ideas, and try new approaches to achieving your health and wellness goals. Instead of fearing change, embrace it as an opportunity for growth, learning, and self-discovery.

➤ Stay Connected: Stay connected to your inner wisdom and intuition, trusting yourself to make choices that align with your values and support your well-being. Tune into your body's signals and listen to what it's telling you about your needs, preferences, and limitations. Stay connected to your inner guidance and let it be your compass on your health journey.

➤ Certainly! Here are some additional tips for building a supportive environment and mindset for long-term success from a personal viewpoint:

➤ Practice Self-Reflection: Take time to reflect on your progress, challenges, and successes on your health and wellness journey. Set aside regular moments for self-reflection, whether it's journaling, meditation, or quiet contemplation, and ask yourself questions like "What am I proud of?" and "What can I learn from this experience?" Use self-reflection as an opportunity for growth and self-discovery, and allow it to guide your actions and decisions moving forward.

➤ Surround Yourself with Inspiration: Surround yourself with sources of inspiration and motivation that remind you of your goals and aspirations. Create a vision board with images, quotes, and affirmations that resonate with you, and display it in a prominent place where you'll see it every day. Fill your social media feeds with accounts and content that uplift and inspire you, and seek out books, podcasts, and other resources that nourish your mind and soul.

➤ Practice Resilience: Cultivate resilience in the face of challenges and setbacks, and view them as opportunities for growth and learning. Instead of viewing obstacles as roadblocks, see them as stepping stones on your journey to success. Practice resilience by staying flexible, adapting to change, and bouncing back from adversity with grace and determination.

➤ Set Healthy Boundaries: Set healthy boundaries to protect your time, energy, and well-being, and prioritize activities and relationships that support your health goals. Learn to say no to things that drain your energy or detract from your priorities, and don't be afraid to enforce boundaries to safeguard your physical, emotional, and mental health. By setting healthy boundaries, you create space for the things that truly matter to you and cultivate a supportive environment for long-term success.

➤ Find Joy in the Journey: Find joy in the journey of self-discovery and personal growth, and celebrate the process of becoming the best version of yourself. Embrace the ups and downs of life with curiosity and enthusiasm, and find moments of joy, gratitude, and wonder in each day. Cultivate a sense of playfulness and adventure, and approach life with an open heart and a positive attitude.

➤ Connect with Nature: Spend time connecting with nature and tapping into its healing and rejuvenating powers. Take regular walks in nature, spend time gardening or tending to plants, or simply sit outside and soak up the sights, sounds, and sensations of the natural world. Nature has a way of grounding us, reducing stress, and fostering a sense of peace and well-being, making it an essential component of a supportive environment for long-term success.

➤ Practice Forgiveness: Practice forgiveness towards yourself and others, releasing any resentment, anger, or negativity that weighs you down. Let go of past mistakes and regrets, and forgive yourself for any perceived failures or shortcomings. Similarly, forgive others for any harm they may have caused you, freeing yourself from the burden of resentment and allowing space for healing and growth.

➤ Stay Curious and Open-Minded: Stay curious and open-minded on your health and wellness journey, exploring new ideas, perspectives, and approaches to living your best life. Be willing to challenge your beliefs and assumptions, and approach each day with a sense of wonder and possibility. By staying curious and open-minded, you'll continue to grow and evolve on your journey towards long-term success.

➤ Celebrate Progress, Not Perfection: Celebrate your progress and achievements, no matter how small, and acknowledge the effort and dedication it took to get there. Instead of striving for perfection, focus on progress and improvement over time, recognizing that every step forward brings you closer to your goals. Celebrate your victories, learn from your setbacks, and keep moving forward with confidence and determination.

➤ Trust Yourself: Trust yourself and your instincts, and believe in your ability to create the life you desire. Trust that you have the strength, resilience, and wisdom to overcome any obstacle and achieve your goals. Listen to your inner voice, follow your intuition, and trust that you're on the right path, even when the way forward may seem uncertain. By trusting yourself, you cultivate a supportive environment and mindset for long-term success, knowing that you have everything you need to thrive.

These tips into your life, you can build a supportive environment and mindset that empowers you to achieve your health and wellness goals for the long term. Remember that building a supportive environment and mindset is a journey, not a destination, and it's okay to take it one step at a time. Stay committed to your vision, trust in yourself, and embrace the journey with courage, resilience, and optimism.

◆ ◆ ◆

CONCLUSION

Summary of the key takeaways from the book "Weight Loss: Culinary Solutions for Sustainable Weight Management" from a personal viewpoint:

➤ Understanding Your Body: The book helps you understand the science behind weight loss, including how calories, metabolism, and nutrition play crucial roles in managing weight effectively. It clears up common misconceptions, empowering you with accurate information to make informed decisions.

➤ Building Healthy Habits: You'll learn the importance of building healthy eating habits, focusing on balanced nutrition, portion control, and mindful eating. The book provides practical strategies and recipes to help you enjoy flavorful meals while reducing calorie intake.

➤ Exploring Culinary Solutions: With a variety of recipes for every meal, the book makes it easy to enjoy delicious, nutritious food that supports your weight loss goals. From breakfasts to snacks and treats, each recipe is designed to keep you satisfied and energized throughout the day.

➤ Meal Planning Made Easy: You'll discover tips and techniques for meal planning and preparation, making healthy eating more convenient and accessible. Whether it's grocery shopping, batch cooking, or meal prepping, the book guides you through the process step by step.

➤ Incorporating Physical Activity: Alongside healthy eating, the book emphasizes the importance of incorporating physical activity into your daily routine for sustainable weight management. It offers practical tips to help you stay active and motivated.

➤ Overcoming Challenges: You'll learn how to overcome common challenges and obstacles on your weight loss journey, from plateaus to motivation slumps. The book provides strategies to help you stay focused and resilient, even when faced with setbacks.

➤ Maintaining Long-Term Success: Beyond just losing weight, the book focuses on maintaining long-term success by setting realistic goals, practicing self-compassion, and staying connected to your sources of motivation and inspiration.

➤ Building a Supportive Mindset: Finally, the book emphasizes the importance of building a supportive environment and mindset for long-term success. From surrounding yourself with positivity to practicing self-reflection and finding joy in the journey, it helps you cultivate the mindset needed to achieve your goals.

Overall, *"Weight Loss: Culinary Solutions for Sustainable Weight Management"* offers a holistic approach to weight loss that empowers you to take control of your health and well-being, one delicious meal at a time.

Dear reader,

I want to talk to you like a friend, because embarking on a journey toward sustainable weight management is a big deal, and I'm here to support you every step of the way.

First off, let's acknowledge that deciding to make changes in your life isn't always easy. It takes courage and determination to prioritize your health and well-being, but trust me, it's worth it. I've been there, and I know the challenges you might face, but I also know the incredible sense of empowerment that comes with taking control of your health.

So, let's start by taking a small step together. It doesn't have to be anything drastic; it could be as simple as choosing a healthy meal over fast food, going for a short walk, or even just taking a moment to think about your goals.

Remember, progress doesn't have to be perfect. There will be good days and not-so-good days, but what matters is that you keep moving forward. Believe in yourself and your ability to overcome obstacles, and know that I'm here cheering you on every step of the way.

And guess what? You don't have to do this alone. Reach out to friends, family, or even online communities for support and encouragement. Sharing your journey with others can make all the difference.

So, my friend, let's take that first step together and begin this journey toward sustainable weight management. You've got this, and I'm here to support you every step of the way.

◆ ◆ ◆

ADDITIONAL RESOURCES

Here's a comprehensive list of recommended weight loss books, websites, and support groups to provide you with further guidance and support on your journey toward sustainable weight management:

- ➤ "The Obesity Code" by Dr. Jason Fung: Explores the root causes of obesity and offers evidence-based strategies for weight loss and improved health.

- ➤ "Atomic Habits" by James Clear: Provides practical insights on building and maintaining healthy habits that support long-term weight management.

- ➤ "The Whole30: The 30-Day Guide to Total Health and Food Freedom" by Melissa Hartwig Urban and Dallas Hartwig: Offers a 30-day program focused on resetting your body and transforming your relationship with food.

- ➤ "Eat to Live" by Dr. Joel Fuhrman: Presents a nutrient-dense, plant-based approach to weight loss and optimal health.

- ➤ "Mindless Eating: Why We Eat More Than We Think" by Brian Wansink: Explores the psychology behind our eating habits and offers practical tips for mindful eating.

- ➤ "The Plant-Based Solution" by Joel K. Kahn, MD: Advocates for a plant-based diet as a sustainable and effective approach to weight loss and overall health.

- ➤ "The Mediterranean Diet Weight Loss Solution" by Julene Stassou MS RD: Provides a comprehensive guide to the Mediterranean diet, including recipes and meal plans for weight loss and improved health.

- ➤ "The End of Dieting" by Dr. Joel Fuhrman: Challenges traditional dieting approaches and offers a scientifically-based plan for achieving sustainable weight loss without deprivation.

Websites

- ➤ MyFitnessPal (www.myfitnesspal.com): Offers a popular app and website for tracking food intake, exercise, and weight loss progress. It also features a supportive community forum.

➤   ChooseMyPlate (www.choosemyplate.gov): Provides practical tips, resources, and meal planning tools based on the Dietary Guidelines for Americans.

➤   SparkPeople (www.sparkpeople.com): Offers free weight loss tools, resources, and community support, including meal plans, exercise trackers, and forums.

➤ Healthline (www.healthline.com): Features evidence-based articles, recipes, and resources on weight loss, nutrition, and healthy living.

➤ Mayo Clinic (www.healthline.com): Provides reliable information and practical tips on weight management, fitness, and healthy living from a trusted medical source.

➤   Verywell Fit (www.verywellfit.com): Offers expert-reviewed articles, recipes, and workout plans to support your weight loss and fitness goals.

Support Groups

➤   Weight Watchers (www.weightwatchers.com): Offers a structured program for weight loss and healthy living, including in-person meetings and online support.

➤   Overeaters Anonymous (www.oa.org): Provides support and fellowship for individuals struggling with compulsive eating habits and weight management issues.

➤ TOPS (Take Off Pounds Sensibly) (www.tops.org): Offers support groups and resources for individuals seeking to lose weight and improve their health through education, motivation, and support.

➤ Reddit - r/loseit (www.reddit.com/r/loseit): A supportive online community where members share their weight loss journeys, progress, tips, and encouragement.

➤ Meetup (www.meetup.com): Search for local groups or events focused on weight loss, fitness, and healthy living in your area.

These resources offer a wealth of information, support, and guidance to help you achieve your weight loss goals and maintain a healthy lifestyle for the long term. Remember, it's important to find the resources and support network that resonate with you and align with your individual needs and preferences.